OXFORD MEDICAL PUBLICATIONS

A Handbook of Paediatric Anaesthesia

PAEDIATRIC ADVANCED LIFE
SUPPORT ALGORITHMS ARE
GIVEN ON PAGES 258 to 263

A HANDBOOK OF
Paediatric Anaesthesia

SECOND EDITION

Edited by

Stephen J. Mather

and

David G. Hughes

Sir Humphry Davy Department of Anaesthesia,
Royal Hospital for Sick Children,
Bristol, BS2 8BJ, UK

OXFORD   NEW YORK   TOKYO
OXFORD UNIVERSITY PRESS
1996

Oxford University Press, Walton Street, Oxford OX2 6DR

Oxford   New York
Athens   Auckland   Bangkok   Bombay
Calcutta   Cape Town   Dar es Salaam   Delhi
Kuala Lumpur   Madras   Madrid   Melbourne
Mexico City   Nairobi   Paris   Singapore
Taipei   Tokyo   Toronto
and associated companies in
Berlin Ibadan

Oxford is a trade mark of Oxford University Press

Published in the United States
by Oxford University Press Inc., New York.

A catalogue record for this book is available from the British Library

Library of Congress Cataloging in Publication Data
A handbook of paediatric anaesthesia/edited by Stephen J. Mather and
David G. Hughes. – 2nd ed.
(Oxford medical publications)
Includes bibliographical references and index.
1. Paediatric anaesthesia – Handbooks, manuals, etc.   I. Mather, S.
James.   II. Hughes, David G. (David Graham)   III. Series.
[DNLM: 1. Anesthesia – in infancy & childhood. WO 440 H236 1996]
RD139.H36   1996   617.9′6798–dc20   95–39066

ISBN 0 19 2627147 (Hbk)

Typeset by EXPO Holdings, Malaysia.
Printed in Great Britain by
Bookcraft (Bath) Ltd
Midsomer Norton, Aron

Preface to the first edition

The object in writing this book has been to fulfil the need for a ready reference for trainees, with readily accessible facts. With the recent increase in specialization within anaesthesia, paediatric work may be daunting to many trainees. The consultant anaesthetist who only occasionally practises paediatric anaesthesia may also find something of value within its pages.

It is obviously very difficult to cover every aspect of paediatric anaesthetic practice but we have tried to provide some guiding principles upon which to base sound decisions.

ACKNOWLEDGEMENT

The authors wish to express their sincere thanks to Mrs Ann Bassett and Mrs Jane McLean for excellent secretarial assistance and to the Department of Medical Illustration, Bristol Royal Infirmary.

Bristol   S. J .M.
1996   D. G. H.

*Life is short and the art long; the occasion fleeting;
experience fallacious and judgement difficult.
Hippocrates: Aphorisms*

Contents

Contributors

S. J. MATHER MB, BS, LRCP, MRCS, DRCOG, FRCA.
Consultant Anaesthetist, Bristol Royal Hospital for Sick Children and Sir Humphry Davy Department of Anaesthesia, Bristol Royal Infirmary; and Honorary Clinical lecturer, University of Bristol.

D. G. HUGHES MD, FRCA.
Consultant Anaesthetist, Bristol Royal Hospital for Sick Children and Sir Humphry Davy Department of Anaesthesia, Bristol Royal Infirmary; and Honorary Clinical Lecturer, University of Bristol.

J. W. O'HIGGINS MB, BS, D Obst. RCOG, FRCA.
Consultant Anaesthetist, Bristol Royal Hospital for Sick Children and Sir Humphry Davy Department of Anaesthesia, Bristol Royal Infirmary; and Honorary Clinical Lecturer, University of Bristol.

S. N. C. BOLSIN MB, BS, FRCA.
Consultant Anaesthetist, Sir Humphry Davy Department of Anaesthesia, Bristol Royal Infirmary; and Honorary Clinical Lecturer, University of Bristol.

C. R. MONK MB, BS, DRCOG, DA, FRCA.
Consultant Anaesthetist, Sir Humphry Davy Department of Anaesthesia, Bristol Royal Infirmary; and Honorary Clinical Lecturer, University of Bristol.

J. I. ALEXANDER MB, BS, LRCP, MRCS, D Obst. RCOG, FRCA.
Consultant Anaesthetist, Sir Humphry Davy Department of Anaesthesia, Bristol Royal Infirmary; and Honorary Clinical Lecturer, University of Bristol.

1

Anatomy and physiology

S. J. Mather

There are differences between preterm and full term babies and the larger child which must be borne in mind. The first few months of life are a period when profound changes in the major systems are taking place. As a consequence, neonates and infants cannot be viewed as smaller versions of the adult or even of the larger child. Each patient must be assessed according to his age and weight. In neonates, any degree of prematurity together with the presence of congenital abnormalities, must be taken into account. In neonates and small infants, the head and abdomen are large in comparison with the rest of the body and the muscles weak.

THE RESPIRATORY SYSTEM

Infants under the age of 6 weeks are obligate nose-breathers. A simple congenital anomaly such as choanal atresia may result in severe respiratory distress.

- The large head and short neck, together with the relatively large tongue in a baby can all make maintaining the airway and intubating a baby difficult for the beginner. Enlarged adenoids may compound the partial obstruction of the airway by the tongue.

- A roll of towel or a small sandbag should be placed under the shoulders and the jaw lifted forward with a finger behind the mandible. The airway must be maintained with the fingers supporting only bony structures. Pressure on the soft tissues in the floor of the mouth will only increase the obstruction.

The thorax is relatively small and the ribs articulate more at right angles with the spine than in the older child and the intercostal muscles are weak. This means that ventilation is largely diaphragmatic.

Distended stomach or bowel will interfere with respiration by hindering diaphragmatic excursion.

- The stomach should always be emptied as much as possible prior to anaesthesia and any ventilated neonate should have a gastric tube *in situ*.

The epiglottis is relatively large, v-shaped, and floppy. It is attached to the inner surface of the anterior thyroid cartilage and along the base of the tongue. The epiglottis is not essential for swallowing[1] and it does not completely close the glottis during the swallowing process.

The larynx

In young children, the larynx lies higher and more anteriorly in the neck, opposite the interspace between the 4th and 5th cervical vertebrae (Fig. 1.1). Attached to the posterolateral surfaces of the cricoid cartilage are the inferior cornua of the thyroid cartilage (Fig. 1.2).

The vocal cords join the anterior vocal processes of the arytenoids to the thyroid cartilage. Ligaments attach the laryngeal cartilages to each other and to the superior cornua of the thyroid cartilage. The pharyngeal constrictor muscles and 'strap' muscles support the larynx.

Complex sliding and rotational movements occur at the crico-arytenoid joints (Fig. 1.3). The posterior crico-arytenoid muscles open the glottis by moving the arytenoids laterally apart. The opposite action is achieved by

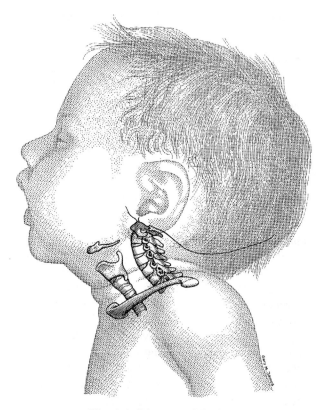

Fig. 1.1 Diagram of the larynx.

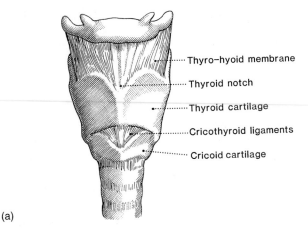

(a)

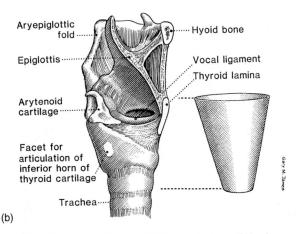

(b)

Fig. 1.2 (a) Anterior view of the larynx; (b) Lateral view of the larynx with thyroid lamina excised.

crico-arytenoid lateralis, the interarytenoids, and thyro-arytenoids, assisted by the cricothyroids, which pull the thyroid cartilage forward, therefore lengthening the cords. All these intrinsic muscles are supplied by the recurrent laryngeal nerve, with the exception of the cricothyroid muscles which are supplied by the superior laryngeal nerve. Both these nerves are branches of the vagus.

In small children the larynx is conical in shape (Fig. 1.2) and the narrowest part of the upper airway is not at the vocal cords but at the level of the cricoid ring. As the child grows, this ring increases in size faster than the trachea, and at 8 or 10 years of age reaches the adult pattern.

The infant larynx is particularly susceptible to oedema formation, even after mild trauma, which can result in marked narrowing and increased airway resistance. The upper airway may be further narrowed by large tonsils and adenoids.

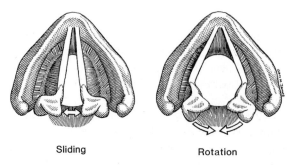

Sliding   Rotation

Fig. 1.3 Movement of the arytenoid cartilages.

The trachea

The full-term neonatal trachea is 4 cm long. Airflow in the trachea is mainly laminar but it becomes more turbulent in the lower trachea and the bronchial orifices. The tracheobronchial angles are similar to those in adults, (30° on the right and 45° on the left). Normally, the larynx and trachea account for only a small part of airflow resistance, but this may be greatly increased in tracheomalacia and subglottic stenosis where a high resistance may be encountered, even during quiet breathing.

The tendency towards the collapse of the trachea during inspiration is resisted both by the cricoid cartilage in the neck and by the negative intrapleural pressure inside the thorax. The trachea and major bronchi collapse during coughing, thus resulting in very high airflow velocities along the major bronchi and trachea. Coughing, however, is relatively ineffective in expelling secretions in the intrapulmonary airways[1] due to their overall large cross-sectional area. Damage to ciliated epithelia, by dry inspired gas, infection, or drugs, may result in reduced mucus clearance.

Tracheal smooth muscle is attached to the posterior ends of the tracheal cartilages, thereby forming the posterior tracheal wall. Experiments in dogs suggest that when smooth muscle tone is decreased, the posterior wall may invaginate and reduce the area of the tracheal lumen.[2] Constriction of this muscle may narrow the lumen, but it does not occlude it. However, constriction of bronchial smooth muscle may totally occlude the bronchial lumen.[2]

Reflexes

Vagal reflexes, which are well known to cause laryngospasm and bradycardia, also affect the lower airways. Bronchospasm and decreased compliance may be precipitated by the presence of an endotracheal tube causing laryngeal stimulation.[3] Resistance to airflow in the larynx may be increased by hypoxia or hypercapnia.[4]

The lungs

The number of generations of bronchi do not increase after birth. However there is increased formation of alveoli postnatally, and true alveoli become apparent by 8 weeks of age. The lung structure becomes similar to that of the adult, comprising approximately 3 million alveoli by the age of 8 years.

At birth, about 2.8 m^2 of alveolar surface is available for gas exchange and this area rises to 12 m^2 at 1 year and 32 m^2 in the 8 year old. The increase in alveolar surface area parallels that of body surface area.

Postnatal lung growth is affected by two major factors: firstly, the space into which the lung can grow (for example, pneumonectomy is followed by compensatory growth in the other lung); and secondly, the inspired oxygen concentration. Experiments in rats have shown that alveolar growth is stimulated by chronic hypoxia and depressed by hyperoxia.

Infants have a high metabolic rate and consequently an increased ventilatory requirement, with respiratory rates of 30 or more breaths per minute in the first year of life. The functional residual capacity as a proportion of total lung volume is small soon after birth but increases throughout infancy. Consequently, when artificial airways are in use, continuous positive airway pressure (CPAP) is beneficial, particularly when nitrogen in the lungs has been washed out, thereby removing its splinting effect upon the alveoli.

Lung volume per unit body weight is similar in infants to that in the older child. When compliance is related to unit lung volume, its value in the infant is also similar. Compliance is, however, generally measured as the combined values of chest wall and lung. Chest wall compliance in the newborn and small infants is very high. The increase in lung volume caused by positive airway pressure reduces alveolar collapse and increases lung compliance. Compliance is decreased by lung disorders such as the infant respiratory distress syndrome. In infants, the closing volume of the lung is relatively large as a fraction of total lung capacity.

- *Airways closure occurs within the tidal range of breathing during anaesthesia with spontaneous respiration unless CPAP is applied.*

In infants the dead space/tidal volume ratio (V_D/V_T) of 1/3 is similar to that in older children and adults. However, because of the infant's small tidal volume, any added apparatus dead space will become significant.

Babies have:
large head
big abdomen
small chest
high O_2 consumption
active reflexes

RESPIRATORY GAS EXCHANGE

Oxygen diffuses down a concentration gradient from a partial pressure in the alveolus of about 110 mm Hg (14.7 kPa) to achieve a pulmonary venous PO_2 of 100 mm Hg (13.3 kPa). As in adults, ventilation–perfusion (V/Q) relationships in children influence the uptake of oxygen. Carbon dioxide is much more diffusible than oxygen and is therefore affected to a lesser extent.

In the adult standing erect, the apices of the lung are relatively better ventilated than the bases, which are over-perfused in relation to the apices. In small children the situation is thought to be less significant, possibly due to the higher pulmonary arterial pressure and the smaller effect of pooling in the bases of the lungs. Any tendency to reduction in lung volume in small children will bring about airway closure and increase V/Q mismatch. Large shunts may occur, with consequent arterial desaturation. Children with such large shunts fail to demonstrate the normal rise in arterial PO_2 during 100 per cent oxygen breathing, as in the hyperoxia test. Shunts do not normally lead to a rise in PCO_2 because small rises in PCO_2 stimulate chemoreceptor drive, thereby increasing ventilation. However, most significant shunts are extrapulmonary and are usually the result of cardiac anomalies.

OXYGEN TRANSPORT

Only a very small fraction of the total oxygen carried in the blood is dissolved in the plasma (0.3 ml dl^{-1} at 100 mm Hg). Most is bound to haemoglobin, each gram of haemoglobin being combined with 1.34 ml of oxygen.

A low arterial PO_2 may be the result of:

- a low inspired PO_2 such as an hypoxic anaesthetic gas mixture;
- hypoventilation;
- ventilation–perfusion mismatch;
- intracardiac or intrapulmonary shunting;
- a reduction in the diffusing capacity of the lung (alveolar–capillary block). In this situation, pulmonary capillary blood does not equilibrate with the alveolar gas during the transit time of the red cell through the capillary.

The oxygen dissociation curve of haemoglobin

This curve represents the change in saturation of haemoglobin in relation to the partial pressure of oxygen in the blood (see Fig. 1.4). For normal adult-type haemoglobin (HbA) a PO_2 of 100 mm Hg (13.3 kPa) represents 97 per cent saturation. The mixed venous values are 40 mm Hg (5.3 kPa) and 75 per cent respectively. Above 60 mm Hg (8.0 kPa), the curve becomes

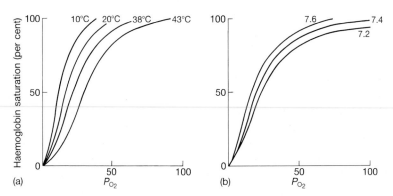

Fig. 1.4 Effects of (a) temperature and (b) pH change on the oxyhaemoglobin dissociation curve.

flattened and increased changes in PO_2 cause only very small changes in
saturation. The affinity of haemoglobin for oxygen is described by the P_{50}
value. For normal adult haemoglobin, at 37 °C and a pH of 7.4, saturation is
50 per cent at about 27 mm Hg (3.6 kPa). The affinity for oxygen increases
as the pH rises; this is known as the Bohr effect. A similar effect occurs with
decreasing temperature and decreasing PO_2. These effects cause a 'left shift'
of the dissociation curve. Opposite changes cause a 'right shift'.

The affinity of haemoglobin for oxygen is also markedly affected by the
concentration of 2,3-disphosphoglycerate (2,3-DPG). This organic phosphate binds with deoxyhaemoglobin but not with oxyhaemoglobin. Increased
levels of 2,3-DPG cause an increase in P_{50} (decreased affinity) and a 'right
shift' in the curve. The effect of this change is to facilitate unloading of
oxygen in the tissues. The amount of 2,3-DPG in stored blood is reduced.
This may be important during massive transfusion because the ability of the
transfused haemoglobin to offload oxygen may be impaired.

High 2,3-DPG levels are found in infants when the normal haemoglobin
level falls to around 10 g dl^{-1}. Oxygen delivery remains the same as that for
an adult with a haemoglobin level of 13 g dl^{-1}, due to the shift in P_{50}[5].

Table 1.1   Haemoglobin — typical values

		Haemoglobin (g dl^{-1})
Neonate	1–7 days	16–20
	1–4 weeks	11–16
	2–3 months	10–12
	1 year	10–12
	5 years	11–13
	12 years	12–14

Table 1.2 Blood volume in relation to body weight

	ml kg^{-1}
Neonate–1 year	80–85
2 years	70
>3 years	60–65

In neonates, with a high proportion of fetal haemoglobin (HbF), the P_{50} is low and the affinity for oxygen is high, due to the poor binding of 2,3-DPG to fetal haemoglobin. This results in a 'left shift' of the dissociation curve and a resulting higher saturation at low PO_2. Fetal haemoglobin still offloads oxygen to the tissues because it is operating over the steep part of the curve.

THE CARDIOVASCULAR SYSTEM

Under normal circumstances, closure of the ductus arteriosus, foramen ovale, and ductus venosus establish the adult pattern of the circulation, with blood flowing through the lungs and returning to the left heart. Failure of normal closure or anatomical imperfections in the cardiac chambers and the great vessels give rise to anomalies which present in early life as congenital heart disease.

Persistent fetal circulation

Pulmonary vascular resistance usually falls rapidly at birth but pulmonary arterial and aortic pressures remain similar until the ductus arteriosus closes, normally within 12 h of birth. The decrease in pulmonary vascular resistance continues throughout the neonatal period. If pulmonary vascular resistance does not decrease shortly after birth, pulmonary hypertension occurs, resulting in a situation which resembles the fetal state with right to left shunting across the ductus arteriosus or patent foramen ovale. This condition is known as 'persistent fetal circulation'.

The neonate has a heart rate of approximately 140 beats min^{-1} but this may vary widely during stress and sleep. The heart gradually decreases throughout infancy and childhood, being about 110–120 beats min^{-1} at 2 years, 100 at 4 years, and 90 at 8 years (see Table 1.3). Heart rates of individuals may vary enormously from these values and still not be of pathological significance. Blood pressure in children was seldom measured in the past, but with modern oscillometric and other methods it can be elicited easily and quickly in all age groups. Systolic blood pressure in the neonate is

Table 1.3 Blood pressure and heart rate — typical values

Age	Blood pressure (mm Hg)		Heart rate (beats min^{-1})
	Systolic	Diastolic	
Neonate	70–80	40–50	120–150
3–6 months	80–90	50–60	120–140
1 year	90–100	60–80	110–130
5 years	95–100	50–80	90–100
12 years	110–120	60–70	80–100

commonly 70–80 mm Hg. This value rises to approximately 90 mm Hg at 2 years and 100 mm Hg between 3 and 6 years (Table 1.3). It gradually assumes the adult value of 110 to 120 mm Hg by teenage. Trends in serial measurements are more important than any one absolute value.

- Infants are particularly prone to bradycardia, frequently associated with a low cardiac output state, if they suffer vagal stimulation such as may occur during laryngoscopy, squint surgery, rectal examination, or traction on peritoneal structures and the processus vaginalis. (Blood pressure measurements may not be meaningful at slow heart rates).

Bradycardia should be treated promptly. Young children usually respond to reductions in blood pressure, or demands for increased cardiac output, by an increase in heart rate. The ability to increase stroke volume is limited and it is reduced still further by myocardial depressants such as halothane.[6]

THE NERVOUS SYSTEM

At birth the spinal cord extends to the level of the third lumbar vertebra. Differential growth between the cord and the spinal canal results in the cord terminating at the level of the first lumbar vertebra at the age of 12 months. Myelination of the peripheral nerves is incomplete at birth and there is controversy as to whether this influences infant neurological responses, particularly with regard to pain perception and neuromuscular function. Autonomic function is well developed at birth and exaggerated responses, such as vagal bradycardia are often seen.

The fontanelles can be used to gain a crude estimate of raised or lowered intracranial pressure. Ultrasound scanning of the brain can also be performed through the fontanelles. Measurement of the size of the fontanelles is of little use because size varies widely in normal babies. Growth in size of the head occurs even if the fontanelles are closed. The rate of closure is not dependent on bone age.[7]

Cerebral blood flow

In the older child or adult, cerebral autoregulation maintains cerebral perfusion relatively constant despite wide variations in systemic blood pressure. In the immature brain there is a deficiency of the muscle layer in cerebral arterioles, impairing the ability of the neonatal brain, especially in the premature, to cope with hypercarbia or hypoxia, so that cerebral blood flow then becomes more pressure-passive, varying with the systemic blood pressure.

Falls in systemic blood pressure are associated with moderate decreases in cerebral perfusion pressure (mean blood pressure minus intracranial pressure) and may result in cerebral injury. In term neonates this is most likely in the parasaggital regions of cerebral cortex but the most vulnerable areas in the premature baby are in the periventricular white matter.[8]

Intracranial haemorrhage

Intracranial haemorrhage may occur in up to 40 per cent of premature neonates. This high incidence may reflect improved survival of very low-birth-weight infants (less than 1000 g). In the premature neonate bleeding occurs from vessels in the subependymal germinal matrix and most suffer associated intraventricular haemorrhage (IVH). A few babies go on to develop infarction of periventricular areas of the brain. Such bleeding is easily detected by ultrasound scan which is routinely performed on premature neonates in the first week of life. In ventilated neonates, the use of muscle relaxants results in a more stable cerebral blood flow and reduced incidence of IVH.

In managing these infants care must be taken to minimize abrupt rises in blood pressure such as occur with endotracheal suction.

THE LIVER

The liver is supplied with blood from both the hepatic artery (25%) and the portal vein (75%). Some synthesis of the bile acids takes place in the fetal liver and this gradually increases throughout pregnancy. The newborn however still possesses only a small synthetic capacity compared with the older child or adult.

The neonate has a much reduced capacity for oxidation, reduction, hydrolysis, or conjugation of drugs due to immaturity of the enzyme systems required. Distribution and binding of drugs is also affected due to the lower albumin, glycoprotein, and lipoprotein levels (see Chapter 2).

METABOLISM, FLUID, AND ELECTROLYTE BALANCE

Metabolism in the neonate

At birth the newborn baby is subjected to considerable cold stress resulting in an increased requirement for heat production. A rise in arterial PO_2 and stress hormone levels contribute to the complex metabolic changes which take place at birth. In full term infants blood glucose falls in the first two hours of life but then rises again. There is an increase in plasma free fatty acids, glycerol, and ketones. Administration of exogenous glucose reduces lipolysis.

Oxygen requirement increases markedly after delivery, reflecting cold stress and stabilizes out at 6–8 ml kg^{-1} in a neutral thermal environment. Thyroid hormones stimulate metabolism of brown fat via non-shivering thermogenesis (see below). Gluconeogenesis is probably active within two hours of birth if the infant is fasted, and most energy production comes from oxidation of free fatty acids which are released at birth.[9]

Neonates, however, are usually put to the breast or fed by other means shortly after birth. The full term neonate possesses greater energy stores than the premature baby who is at considerable risk from hypoglycaemia, particularly during cold stress. Long-term starvation results in hypernatraemia and hyperbilirubinaemia. Administration of glucose reduces lipolysis and circulating levels of free fatty acids.

Premature infants do not have such precise regulatory mechanisms for glucose as the full-term baby and may equally well develop hyperglycaemia when given intravenous glucose. Very low-birth-weight infants are particularly prone to this.[10] It has been shown recently that only small quantities of exogenous glucose are required to prevent hypoglycaemia in the older child peroperatively.[11] Stress-related insulin antagonism does not then result in hyperglycaemia, as sometimes occurs when 10% glucose is given intraoperatively to older children.

The renal system

At birth the glomeruli are similar in number to those of adults. Changes in the microscopic structure continue into teenage. The infant kidney, although adequate for the normal physiological loads placed upon it, responds poorly to certain stresses. It has difficulty in coping with large water loads, sodium loads, and excess hydrogen ions. The ability to concentrate urine is limited. These factors must be borne in mind when assessing fluid requirements perioperatively.

Water and electrolytes

The newborn infant requires much greater care in the assessment of fluid and electrolyte needs compared with the older child when the more mature kidney and associated control systems can compensate for errors to a greater degree. Total body water is about 80 per cent of body weight at term, 45 per cent of which is extracellular water.

Glomerular filtration rate (GFR)

GFR is very low in the premature infant. This may be due to the fact that glomerulogenesis is incomplete before 34 weeks gestation. Even in the full term neonate it remains low, probably because the glomerulus continues to develop functionally after birth. At birth, renal vascular resistance decreases and blood flow increases markedly. GFR increases in proportion to gestational age. (GFR will, however, fall if the infant is dehydrated or has a low cardiac output, e.g. from hypoxia.) Following completion of glomerulogenesis at 34 weeks gestation, GFR increases linearly as related to surface area up to the age of 1 year. This is thought to be due to morphological changes in the glomerulus and increasing renal blood flow. GFR is approximately 30 ml min^{-1} (1.73 m^{-2}) on day one, 70 at 3 months, and 105–110 from 2 years onwards.[12]

More than 1 ml kg^{-1} h^{-1} is regarded as an adequate urine flow in the perioperative period. Insensible water loss is high in the neonate and extremely high in the premature infant (in excess of 75 g m^{-2} hour^{-1} at 26 weeks gestation). Radiant heat increases transepidermal water loss dramatically.[13] It is therefore important to maintain high ambient humidity for the premature infant. This can be done by wrapping the infant's limbs and covering him with plastic sheeting before exposure to radiant heat.

Provision of free water (in the form of glucose solution) of about 80 ml per 100 calories metabolized allows for the high insensible losses and reduced renal concentrating ability of the neonate. Older children behave more like adults and with a smaller turnover of water, require less fluid maintenance. Resuscitation of small infants when they suffer profound derangements of circulating volume (e.g. intestinal obstruction) or are septic is particularly challenging.

Perioperative fluid maintenance requirements are given on pp. 94–5.

Electrolyte requirements

Very premature infants are unable to conserve sodium and require considerable supplementation (up to 9–10 mM kg^{-1} day^{-1}),[14] neither are they able to tolerate a sodium load very well. Although aldosterone secretion is increased in the newborn, the physiological response is less than in older children. The full term neonate is adequately supplied by 1.5 mM kg^{-1} day^{-1} which increases to 2–3 mM kg^{-1} day^{-1} after 2 postnatal weeks. Potassium requirements are 2 mM kg^{-1} day^{-1} in neonates. Older children require less, but 2 mM kg^{-1} day^{-1} at all ages supplies the body's needs and does not present an undue load. Chloride mirrors the potassium requirements.

Acid–base balance

The newborn infant has a limited ability to excrete hydrogen ions. However even ex-premature babies develop a much greater capacity for excretion of acid loads after a few weeks. The neonate has a reduced ability to conserve bicarbonate in the renal tubules. This results in a lower plasma pH (7.3–7.4). The plasma bicarbonate is low (18–22 mM litre^{-1}). Phosphate and ammonia excretion are reduced in the first week of life and so the amount of buffer available in the urine is less. This limits the neonate's ability to excrete an acid load.

TEMPERATURE REGULATION

Babies have a large surface area relative to their weight and tend to lose body heat quickly. They have little body fat and are thus not well insulated. This effect is exacerbated during anaesthesia when radiant heat losses may be high and metabolic heat production minimal. The inhalation of dry anaesthetic gases further increases heat loss due to the latent heat of vaporization which needs to be supplied to humidify the inspired gas.

The infant's ability to regulate his temperature is less well developed than that of the adult. The oxygen cost for maintaining body temperature is minimal at skin-to-air temperature gradients of between 2 and 4 °C. A 'neutral thermal environment' will normally be between 32 and 34 °C. To maintain thermal equilibrium, heat production must equal heat loss.

Factors affecting heat production

- Basal metabolic rate (thyroid disease, infection, drugs).
- Increase in muscular activity.
- Non-shivering thermogenesis (β-adrenergic receptor-mediated increase in metabolism of fatty acids and glucose). This may include the metabolism of brown fat, although its significance in humans is debatable.[15,16]

Non-shivering thermogenesis is abolished by β-blockade.[17] Glucocorticoids and thyroxine are also thought to play a part in the control of this response.[18, 19] Non-shivering thermogenesis is the more important of these mechanisms in children under 6 months of age.

Induced hypothermia

Induced hypothermia forms part of certain anaesthetic techniques, as for example in cardiac surgery. Provided homeostatic mechanisms are allowed to function, cooling initially increases oxygen consumption, but then it falls as core temperature is reduced. In lightly anaesthetized infants, the increase in oxygen demand may be more than the baby can cope with, thereby leading to hypoglycaemia, hypoxaemia, and acidosis. The extent to which anaesthetic agents affect the regulatory responses is not clear. Hypothermia is a potent cause of apnoea in small babies, particularly during recovery from anaesthesia.

Neonates
Have reduced capacity to handle drugs
May be prone to apnoea
Need care with fluid balance
Easily get cold

REFERENCES

1. Proctor, D. F. (*1977*). The upper airways II. The larynx and trachea. *American Review of Respiratory Disease*, **115**, 315.
2. Murtagh, P. S. *et al.* (1971). Bronchial mechanics in excised dog lobes. *Journal of Applied Physiology*, **31**, 403.
3. Olsen, C. R., de Kock, M. A., and Colebatch, H. J. H. (1967). Stability of airways during reflex bronchoconstriction, *Journal of Applied Physiology*, **23**, 23.
4. Dixson, M. *et al.* (1974). Studies on laryngeal calibre during stimulation of peripheral and central chemoreceptors, pneumothorax and increased respiratory loads. *Journal of Physiology*, **236**, 347.
5. Card, R. T. and Brain, M. C. (1973). The 'anaemia' of childhood. Evidence for a physiologic response to hyperphosphataemia. *New England Journal of Medicine*, **288**, 388.
6. Barash, P. G. *et al.* (1978). Ventricular function in children during halothane anaesthesia: an echocardiographic evaluation. *Anaesthesiology*, **49**, 79.
7. Duc, G. and Largo, R. H. (1986). Anterior fontanel: size and closure in term and pre-term infants. *Paediatrics*, **78**, 904.
8. Avery, G. B., Fletcher, M. A., and Macdonald, M. G. (eds) (1994). *Neonatology: Pathophysiology and management of the newborn* p. 1124. J. B. Lippincot Co. Philadelphia.
9. Kalhan, S., Savin, S., and Adam, P. (1976). Measurement of glucose turnover in the human newborn with glucose-1-^{13}C. *Journal of Clinical Endocrinology and Metabolism*, **43**, 704.
10. Dweck, H. and Cassady, G. (1974). Glucose intolerance in infants of very low birth weight I. Incidence of hyperglycaemia in infants of birth weights 1100 gms or less. *Paediatrics*, **53**, 189.
11. Dubois, C., Gouyet, L., Murat, I. *et al.* (1992). Lactated Ringer with 1% dextrose: an appropriate solution for peri-operative fluid therapy in chidren. *Paediatric Anaesthesia*, **2**, 99.
12. Roy, L. P. (1973). Renal physiology in children. *Anaesthesia and Intensive Care*, **1**, 453.

13. Baumgart, S., Engle, W. D., Fox, W. W. *et al.* (1981). Effective heat shielding on convective and evaporative heat losses and radiant heat transfer in the premature infant. *Journal of Paediatrics*, **99**, 948.

14. Engelke, S. C., Shar, B. L. *et al.* (1978). Sodium balance in very low birth weight infants. *Journal of Paediatrics*, **93**, 837.

15. Schiff, E. L., Stern, L., and Ledue, J. (1966). Chemical thermogenesis in newborn infants; catecholamine excretion and the plasma non-esterified fatty acid response to cold exposure. *Paediatrics*, **37**, 577.

16. Stern, L., Lees, M. H., and Ledue, J. (1965). Environmental temperature, oxygen consumption and catecholamine excretion in newborn infants. *Paediatrics*, **36**, 367.

17. Silverman, W. *et al.* (1964). Warm nape of the newborn. *Paediatrics*, **33**, 984.

18. Jenssen, K. (1980). Relation between thyroid function and human non-shivering thermogenesis. *Acta Anaethesiologica Scandinavica*, **24**, 144.

19. Jenssen, K. (1980). Cortisol fluctuations in plasma in relation to human regulatory non-shivering thermogenesis. *Acta Anaesthesiologica Scandinavica*, **24**, 151.

2

Pharmacology

S. J. Mather and J. I. Alexander

GENERAL PHARMACOLOGY

There is a marked difference in the way a small infant copes with a drug load compared with the older child or adult.[1,2]

Absorption

Absorption is generally less important than distribution since, apart from premedication and post-operative analgesia, drugs in anaesthetic practice are usually given parenterally. The volatile agents are of course the exception.

Most orally administered drugs are absorbed only after entering the small intestine. The rate of gastric emptying is therefore important. Most are not actively transported and reach the portal circulation by diffusion. Many are subject to first pass metabolism by the liver. The neonatal gastric juice is less acidic than in older children and adults, which may affect the ionization and bioavailability of some drugs.

Transdermal absorption is more rapid through the well perfused thin epidermis of infants than through the more keratinized skin of adults. Thus absorption of a dose of EMLA or amethocaine cream in a given time is partly inversely proportional to age. The uptake of transdermal fentanyl through the skin is also increased.

Distribution

This encompasses the dilution of the drug in body water and its subsequent delivery to sites within the body. Factors which affect this distribution are:

- water v. lipid solubility;
- blood flow;
- protein binding (intra- and extravascular);
- the presence of other drugs competing for specific and non-specific binding sites;

- pH. The rate of transfer across membranes, e.g. into the brain, is related to the degree of ionization and therefore differs from the adult because of the lower pH.

Protein binding is less in neonates than in older children and adults. This reflects their lower albumin levels, higher bilirubin concentration, and lower pH. There is thus a larger apparent distribution volume, weight for volume.[3]

Acid drugs such as barbiturates bind mostly to albumin, whereas basic drugs, e.g. morphine bind more to globulin, lipoproteins, and glycoproteins. Local anaesthetic agents may achieve a higher free fraction in the neonate due to lower levels of alpha$_1$ acid glycoprotein.

Blood flow to organs per unit weight is variable with age, neonates having a relatively smaller muscle mass.[4] The cardiac output at birth is about 200 ml kg^{-1} min^{-1} reaching about 100 ml kg^{-1} min^{-1}. Rapid circulation times in babies result in faster distribution of drugs.

The larger blood volume and total body water per kilogram also affects the final concentration delivered to the receptor site or target organ. Thus, larger doses per unit body weight need to be given to neonates and infants to achieve the same final concentration. It must be remembered, however, that additional receptor sensitivity may exist to some drugs, for example non-depolarizing muscle relaxants. Redistribution into fat is also variable with age, reflecting the relative proportion of muscle fat and total body water.

Excretion

Most drugs used in anaesthesia undergo some biotransformation before excretion. Only small, ionized molecules, easily filtered and not reabsorbed by the kidney or excreted only via the lung (such as nitrous oxide), remain unchanged. Anaesthetic drugs in general tend to be rather fat soluble and are highly protein bound.

Such compounds need to be converted by the body into more water soluble chemicals which can be renally excreted. Some of this chemical change may take place in the lung or intestine, or simply by hydrolysis in the plasma, but most is achieved by the liver. Metabolites are often inactive but some possess similar properties to the parent compound (benzodiazepines) or are toxic in their own right (cyanide; norpethidine). Sometimes the process of metabolism converts a less or inactive drug to a more active metabolite (diamorphine; prednisone).

Metabolism may consist of rendering the drug water soluble by, for example, hydroxylation or by conjugation with another substance such as glucuronic acid, sulphate, or an amino acid. These two processes may, in fact be sequential (phase I and phase II reaction). The enzymes required to catalyse these reactions e.g. mixed oxidase or cytochrome P450 and glucoronyl transferase, may be deficient or absent in the neonate especially the premature. The exception is hydrolysis, which is usually normal. Adequate phase II pathways have usually developed by 3 months of age, although metabolism of morphine, for example, may not reach adult levels until after 60 weeks post-conceptual age.

Polar compounds produced by metabolism are subsequently excreted via the kidney. This may be by simple filtration or by active transport such as occurs with glucuronides. The elimination half-life is much reduced for many drugs in the newborn period. This is related to lower glomerular filtration rates (GFR) and tubular secretion. For practical purposes, GFR can be assumed to equal adult values at 3 months and tubular secretion by 6 months of age.

So far, we have considered the effects of physiological differences on the general pharmacology of parenterally administered drugs.

For volatile agents, the main considerations must be the blood-gas solubility of the agent, alveolar ventilation (which may be increasingly depressed by the agent), cardiac output, and regional blood flow. Right to left intracardiac shunts and ventilation/perfusion (V/Q) mismatch may significantly prolong the uptake of gaseous agents.[5] Increased pulmonary or decreased systemic vascular resistance may reverse left to right shunts. Alveolar ventilation is much higher on a weight basis in small children, wash-in and wash-out of gases being more rapid.[6,7] Although blood-solubility differs with age,[8] the precise reasons for the differences are not yet known. Uptake of halothane has, however, been shown to be more rapid than in adults due to decreased solubility. The clinical effect of volatile agents is further augmented by the greater proportion of cardiac output which is directed to the vessel-rich group. The blood–brain barrier may also permit enhanced diffusion in the newborn.[9]

VOLATILE ANAESTHETIC AGENTS

The uptake of volatile agent from the lung is dependent upon:

- (P_A-P_V) for the agent, where P_A = alveolar partial pressure and P_V = the mixed venous partial pressure;
- blood-gas solubility;
- cardiac output.

When the volatile agent is first introduced there is a concentration (and partial pressure) gradient from the circuit to the tissues. As the agent is continually being removed from the lung (when P_V is low), uptake is rapid and a high concentration must be given to achieve a satisfactory alveolar partial pressure. As the tissues equilibrate, the partial pressure in the alveolae, blood, and tissues rises. When the vessel-rich group has equilibrated, uptake falls and the inspired concentration can then be reduced. Tissue uptake depends upon blood flow to the tissue, the solubility of the agent in the type of tissue (fat, nerve, muscle), and the arteriolar partial pressure minus the partial pressure of the particular tissue.

For any given tissue there will thus be a rate of uptake which depends upon all these factors. Uptake of hydrocarbon anaesthetics will be high in the brain because it forms part of the 'vessel rich group' with a rich blood supply and a large proportion of lipid.

A large mass of tissue (e.g. fat) which is poorly perfused will have a high capacity to store the volatile agent but it will be cleared most slowly when the inspired agent is discontinued. Total equilibration may take many hours or even days for agents with high fat solubility. Only the initial phases of equilibration with the vessel rich group are important during the induction of anaesthesia with volatile agents. The differences in blood-gas and tissue partition coefficients, fat mass, volume of distribution, alveolar ventilation, and regional blood flow account for the differences in volatile agent uptake between small children and adults. Anaesthetic requirement, as measured by MAC values (minimal alveolar concentration which prevents movement to surgical stimulus in 50 per cent of patients) varies inversely with age.

MAC has been shown to increase over the first few hours of life,[10–12] and this continues throughout the neonatal period. Surprisingly, however, MAC values fall after six months of age. The reason for this is unknown but could be related to the actual delivery concentration or partial pressure at the site of action of volatile agents. A higher partial pressure may be required in the newborn due to the greater water content of the brain. Differences in blood-gas solubility with age may also play a part.[13] MAC is only an *average* value and great variation between patients exists. It seems that newborns in the first few days of life manifest decreased sensitivity to painful stimuli; their ability to cope with large incisions post-operatively in the absence of administered analgesia is well known. The neurophysiological mechanisms underlying this response are as yet unclear but endorphin levels which are known to be elevated at birth fall over the first month of life, as does the receptor population.

INDIVIDUAL INHALATIONAL AGENTS

Nitrous oxide

Nitrous oxide is a simple molecule, a true gas at room temperature. The MAC for nitrous oxide in adults is variously reported at between 105 and 120%. Unless an hypoxic mixture is given, it must be supplemented to achieve '1 MAC' or greater. In the main, nitrous oxide is used in paediatric anaesthesia as:

- a diluent for oxygen;
- to provide some analgesia and reduce the concentration of volatile agent required;
- as the initial induction agent prior to the introduction of volatile agents. The uptake of nitrous oxide by the blood from the lung increases the concentration of volatile agents given concurrently and increases their rate of uptake, 'the second gas effect'. Nitrous oxide has only a slight, sweet smell and is well tolerated, making the introduction of more pungent agents such as isoflurane more acceptable;
- as a sedative agent during procedures under regional anaesthesia.

Because it is rather insoluble in blood, nitrous oxide rapidly achieves equilibrium with the alveolar concentration. This confers upon it the property of rapid induction and recovery. If approximately half the anaesthetic potency of a gas mixture is ascribed to nitrous oxide, faster awakening will occur than if volatile agents are used alone, except in the case of desflurane (see below). Rapid diffusion into the alveolus from the blood may, however, reduce alveolar oxygen concentrations (diffusion hypoxia). High concentrations of oxygen should therefore be given for at least 10 minutes following anaesthesia with nitrous oxide. Because nitrous oxide is a very diffusible gas, it will rapidly equilibrate with any gas-filled body cavity, for example air in the gut or a pneumothorax.

Unlike other inhalational agents, there is minimal potentiation of non-depolarizing muscle relaxants.

Overall, nitrous oxide is a very safe agent. Cardiovascular depression is minimal[14] and there is little change in pulmonary vascular resistance, clearly its use is limited when high inspired oxygen concentrations are required.

One drawback is the potential to cause nausea and many paediatric anaesthetists are now moving away from the use of nitrous oxide, particularly in older children.

Hydrocarbon anaesthetics

This group includes halothane and the halogenated ethers enflurane, isoflurane, desflurane, and sevoflurane. Halogenated agents form the mainstay of paediatric anaesthetic practice. Vast experience with halothane now exists (it was introduced in 1956) but because of the perceived risk of hepatotoxicity, repeat use is declining even in paediatric practice. It is, however, unquestionably the easiest of these agents to use clinically and is unrivalled for smoothness of induction and cost.[15]

Enflurane does not appear to enable even slightly painful procedures to take place until several minutes after the eyelash reflex is lost. Coughing and stridor are more common than with halothane. Theoretically induction or recovery should be more rapid with all the halogenated ethers than with halothane due to their lower blood solubility. Sevoflurane and desflurane are particularly insoluble compared with the others due to halogenation solely with fluorine.[16,17] Desflurane has the lowest blood–tissue partition coefficient of all the volatile agents. This gives rapid equilibration with the inspired concentration and implies fast inhalational induction. However, because desflurane is so pungent, coughing and breath holding preclude rapid rises in the inspiratory concentration limiting its use for inhalational induction of anaesthesia. Irritation of the airway is not a problem during maintenance anaesthesia with desflurane and rapid adjustment to the inspired concentration occurs giving precise control over the depth of anaesthesia. Due to their low solubility, early recovery is faster from anaesthesia with sevoflurane or desflurane than from isoflurane. All the halogenated hydrocarbon anaesthetics depress respiration and the slope of the CO_2 response curve.

In practice, the smooth induction and recovery provided by halothane outweighs many of its disadvantages. A popular technique for inhalational induction is to use a sequential technique, beginning with nitrous oxide and then introducing halothane. When induction is complete, maintenance anaesthesia is provided by the inhalational agent of choice using nitrous oxide and oxygen or oxygen–air as the carrier gas.

Biotransformation of halogenated anaesthetics
Of greater significance when considering possible toxic effects is the degree to which these agents undergo metabolism (see Table 2.1). There are now several reports in the literature claiming halothane induced liver damage in paediatric patients.[18] Biotransformation of halothane in children is not significantly different from that in adults.[19]

Effects on cardiac output
Halothane, enflurane, desflurane, and sevoflurane all reduce cardiac output. There is very little reduction in cardiac output with isoflurane[20] (see Table 2.2). At clinically useful concentration, the fall in blood pressure which occurs with enflurane and halothane is due to myocardial depression without

Table 2.1 Biotransformation of inhalational agents

Agent	Approximate % biotransformation
Nitrous oxide	<0.01
Desflurane	0.02
Isoflurane	0.2
Enflurane	2
Sevoflurane	2
Halothane	20

Table 2.2   Volatile anaesthetic agents — comparison of properties

	Halothane	Enflurane	Isoflurane	Desflurane	Sevoflurane
Myocardial depression	+	+	±	+	+
SVR	±	↓	↓↓	↓	↓
Respiratory depression	+	+++	++	++	++
Rapid recovery	+	++	+++	++++	++++

a concomitant increase in heart rate sufficient to maintain normotension.[21] Both sevoflurane and desflurane depress myocardial contractility. Sevoflurane, like halothane has little effect on heart rate. Desflurane is more like isoflurane and increases heart rate. Enflurane, isoflurane, sevoflurane, and desflurane do not predispose to arrhythmias if adrenaline is used. The use of exogenous adrenaline is contraindicated if halothane is being administered. The fall in blood pressure which occurs when halothane is given is thought to be due to depression of baroreceptor reflexes.[22] Some improvement in blood pressure can be achieved by the administration of anticholinergic drugs but ventricular ejection fraction remains lowered.

Stability in soda lime

With the increasing use of circle systems in paediatric anaesthesia, stability in soda lime is important. Halothane, enflurane, isoflurane, and desflurane are all stable. Sevoflurane, however, is broken down by warm, moist soda lime. Several degradation products have been identified but only one appears to be important clinically and has been termed compound 'A' (1,1,1,3,3,3-pentafluoroisopropenyl fluoromethyl ether). In a study by Frink *et al.*,[16] patients were exposed to 5 MAC-hours of sevoflurane in circle systems using baralyme, which attains a higher temperature than soda-lime. The peak concentration of compound 'A' was 60 parts per million (ppm). (Toxic concentrations in rats were stated as 1050–1090 ppm after 1 hour and 340–490 ppm after 3 hours.) Lethal doses cause renal tubular necrosis and lung congestion.

Renal toxicity due to fluoride ion

Biotransformation of sevoflurane yields free inorganic fluoride ion from the fluoromethyl group. Peak concentrations were about 30 mM l^{-1} after 2 MAC hours.[16] The toxic level in adult humans is said to be 50 mM l^{-1}.

Practical problems

Sevoflurane can be used in a conventional plenum temperature-compensated vaporizer in the same was as halothane, enflurane, and isoflurane. Desflurane, however, has a vapour pressure close to 1 atmosphere at room temperature, boiling at 23.5 °C. Because of the very steep slope of the vapour pressure/temperature curve of desflurane, an electrically heated and thermostatically controlled vaporizer is employed which maintains the agent at 39 °C (e.g. Ohmeda Tec 6).

Effects on systemic vascular resistance

Systemic vascular resistance (SVR) undergoes the most marked fall following the administration of isoflurane. Enflurane and desflurane produce moderate falls in SVR. Sevoflurane does this to a smaller extent and there is hardly any reduction in SVR with halothane. Although peripheral veins 'open up' when all these agents are given, in the case of halothane this produces almost no change in SVR. Changes in SVR when the pulmonary vascular resistance remains little altered, many lead to right to left shunting. This may have serious consequences in those with critical hypoxia or if a bubble of air from an intravenous cannula is allowed to enter the circulation when it may cross a septal defect and cause arterial gas embolization (paradoxical embolus).

INTRAVENOUS ANAESTHETIC AGENTS

The choice lies between the barbiturates methohexitone and thiopentone, di-isopropyl phenol (propofol), ketamine, and etomidate. Benzodiazepines can be employed but are more generally used for sedation rather than induction of unconsciousness.

Thiopentone

In the UK, thiopentone is used as a 2.5% alkaline solution. Since its introduction in 1934, vast experience with this drug has been gained in all types of anaesthesia.

It is very lipid soluble, rapidly crossing the blood–brain barrier. Apnoea is marked after average induction doses (5–6 mg kg^{-1}) but vagal tone is not depressed and laryngeal spasm may easily occur. Cardiac output is reduced, and hypotension may be marked in the presence of hypovolaemia, due to a combination of myocardial depression and peripheral vasodilatation. Asthma is a relative contraindication as bronchospasm may be intense. Recovery from thiopentone is initially due to redistribution, mainly into fat. Plasma protein binding is high and elimination is slow. In adults an elimination half-life of about 12 hours is usually quoted but in children this may be less. There may be considerable postoperative sedation after large or repeated doses.

Methohexitone

Methohexitone, an oxybarbiturate, is still used in adult practice but only rarely in paediatrics. Again solubilized with sodium carbonate it is a strongly alkaline solution used in 1% concentration. 1–2 mg kg^{-1} of body weight is required for induction of anaesthesia. It is more potent weight-for-weight than thiopentone and undergoes more rapid elimination from the body. The elimination half-life is around 3 hours.[23] Residual sedation is less and the drug has been widely used in the past for day case anaesthesia, especially in dentistry.

Disadvantages include breath holding, hiccough, and pain on injection. There is a moderate fall in blood pressure but usually less than after thiopentone. Excitatory movements are usual and may be a nuisance. These can be reduced by the concurrent use of opioid analgesics. Methohexitone may precipitate spike and wave activity on the electroencephalogram.

All barbiturates are contraindicated in acute porphyrias.

Etomidate

Etomidate, an imidazole derivative, has now largely been superseded by propofol. Its main advantage is said to be cardiovascular stability in patients with severe cardiac disease. Its main disadvantage is adrenocortical suppression with repeated doses or infusion and this has been reported after even a single dose. Common undesirable side-effects are pain on injection and excitatory muscle movement, but recovery is rapid. It has only a limited place in paediatric anaesthetic practice.

Propofol

Introduced in 1983, 2,6-di-isopropyl phenol in a lipid emulsion containing soyabean oil, glycerol and egg phosphatide has become a deservedly popular agent in both adult and paediatric practice. Recovery is rapid and superior to methohexitone.[24] Several papers have examined the use of propofol for induction in children.[25,26] Pain on injection is common and can be reduced (although not abolished) by the addition of lignocaine.[27] Various regimens have been tried but 1 to 2 mg of lignocaine per ml of propofol is usually used. For induction of anaesthesia in children up to 3.5 mg kg^{-1} initially is recommended.[26] Propofol is now widely used for short-term (peroperative) infusion in paediatric anaesthesia with good results. It should not be used for intensive care sedation in children. The half-life is context-dependent, that is it is longer after a long infusion than after a short infusion.

Ketamine

Ketamine is described as producing 'dissociative anaesthesia' (dissociation of the cortex from the limbic system). The onset of complete anaesthesia is preceded by intense analgesia, and this persists after consciousness has returned. Indeed, ketamine may be used in subanaesthetic doses for painful procedures, supplemented with other sedative agents, rather than as the sole anaesthetic. Ketamine is said to 'preserve' normal laryngeal reflexes with sufficient muscle tone to allow a minimally obstructed airway, but it must be stressed that this cannot be relied upon and the airway should not be left unsupervised or unmonitored. Ketamine produces intense salivation and should therefore be used in combination with an antisialogogue.

Hallucination and dreaming may occur during recovery from ketamine anaesthesia which can be reduced by the prior administration of benzodiazepines, but retrograde amnesia is not engendered by this manoeuvre. Unpleasant dreaming is said to be less common in children. Nausea and vomiting occurs more frequently than with the other agents previously discussed.

Ketamine causes a rise in blood pressure. Cerebral blood flow is increased and this leads to a concomitant rise in intracranial pressure. Intraocular pressure is increased, although the oculo-cardiac reflex is depressed.

The major indication for the use of this agent is for repeated short painful procedures such as burns dressings, brief radiotherapy, or oncology procedures. It is also suggested for field use after major disasters or in developing countries where anaesthetic facilities are minimal, particularly for children. It is predictably effective when given intramuscularly. Low dose ketamine e.g. $50–100$ μg kg^{-1} is being used increasingly for neuropathic pain e.g. phantom limb pain or in terminal care.

INDUCTION OF ANAESTHESIA BY THE RECTAL ROUTE (BASAL NARCOSIS)

Although not practised to any extent in the UK this technique is popular on the continent of Europe. Thiopentone is usually used in doses of about 50 mg kg^{-1}, of a 4 or 10% solution, although midazolam and methohexitone have been used. The drug is administered via a rectal catheter usually in the ward. Intravenous supplements can be given in the operating theatre. If this method of induction is chosen, the child must be constantly supervised since airway obstruction may easily occur.

BENZODIAZEPINES

Benzodiazepines are widely used for premedication in paediatric practice, particularly diazepam and midazolam. Diazepam in a dose of 1 mg kg^{-1} or midazolam 0.5 mg kg^{-1} to a maximum of 30 mg are suitable for oral administration. Midazolam can be supplied in a stable solution for oral administration but the intravenous preparation diluted in a small amount of fruit juice is also acceptable. Oral midazolam is particularly rapidly acting and children may need to be placed in bed under supervision within 20 minutes of its administration to prevent them falling and injuring themselves. Midazolam has also been given by the nasal route. (0.2 mg kg^{-1}), although this route is less acceptable to the children than the oral route.[28,29]

Benzodiazepine premedication does, however, lead to prolonged recovery from anaesthesia particularly after short procedures and this is significant even after midazolam[30] which is considered to be a short-acting drug.

Although diazepam, midazolam, and flunitrazepam have all been used for induction of anaesthesia, benzodiazepines are now largely used in paediatric anaesthetic practice for sedation with amnesia to cover procedures under local analgesia, as adjuvants during general anaesthesia, and in intensive care.

Diazepam is available in a lipid formulation which reduces the incidence of pain on injection and thrombophlebitis. It is highly protein bound in the plasma. Elimination half-life may be several days in premature neonates but this is reduced in infants to less than 24 h, due principally to maturation of conjugative metabolism. Diazepam is best given in single doses for this reason and because some of its metabolites are active and undergo entero-hepatic recirculation. The clinical effect of even a single dose is therefore unpredictable. Significant respiratory depression may be produced by intravenous administration. The rectal route is used for anticonvulsant therapy and can also be used for basal sedation in the ward.

Unlike diazepam, midazolam is more water soluble. It is highly protein bound. Metabolites do not contribute greatly to its sedative effect as these are rapidly eliminated as water-soluble conjugates. Oxidative metabolism is the principal route of inactivation. The reduced capacity of neonates for this process would suggest a longer elimination time at this age.

Most anaesthetists would consider midazolam unsuitable for induction of anaesthesia since its effects are unpredictable. It may be useful, however, in reducing the dose of other agents required. Minimal depression of cardiovascular function is seen, but clinically significant respiratory depression after $150–200 \ \mu g \ kg^{-1}$ is rare.

Midazolam is commonly used by infusion in intensive care units for sedation and amnesia in ventilated patients, $100–300 \ \mu g \ kg^{-1} \ h^{-1}$ being commonly employed. Infusion rates up to $300 \ \mu g \ kg^{-1} \ h^{-1}$ do not result in cumulation unless liver function is abnormal.

Reversal of benzodiazepine sedation

The effects of both diazepam and midazolam can be adequately but temporarily reversed by flumazenil, a benzodiazepine antagonist. It is, however, very expensive.

MUSCLE RELAXANTS IN PAEDIATRIC ANAESTHESIA

The neuromuscular junction is not mature at birth.[31] Throughout infancy there is an increase in muscle mass as a proportion of body weight and the effect of neuromuscular blocking drugs in terms of dose–response and kinetics varies.

Myelination of nerve fibres continues after birth, conduction velocity thereby increasing and the potential for acetylcholine release at the motor end plate increases with maturity. Even allowing for differences in distribution volume and concomitant anaesthesia, infants appear to display relative resistance to suxamethonium and sensitivity to non-depolarizing neuromuscular blockade.[32,33] Neonates posses a much lower capacity for hydrolysis of suxamethonium than older children or adults but due to the increased volume of extracellular water, a greater dose on a weight-for-weight basis is required in neonates. Although extracellular fluid volume correlates well with surface area, and if doses are given on this basis, relative resistance to suxamethonium is still seen in young infants.[34]

Depolarizing neuromuscular blockade — suxamethonium

Suxamethonium is widely used in paediatric anaesthesia. It produces rapid and profound muscle relaxation when given in adequate dosage (1.5 mg kg^{-1} in neonates and small infants, 1 mg kg^{-1} in older children). Unless preceded by a vagolytic drug such as atropine (20 μg kg^{-1}) or glycopyrronium (10 μg kg^{-1}), bradycardia is very common. Ventricular ectopic beats also occur. Intra-ocular pressure is raised due to contraction of the extra-ocular muscles during fasciculation. Intragastric pressure is increased but lower oesophageal sphincter tone may be also, thereby preserving barrier pressure and not increasing the likelihood of regurgitation.

Serum potassium is said to rise by up to 0.5 mmol l^{-1} in the average patient, but more after spinal injury or in other denervation disorders where muscle damage or wasting has occurred.

Suxamethonium is a known trigger agent for malignant hyperpyrexia.

Non-depolarizing neuromuscular blocking agents (NDPs)

Several studies[35-37] have suggested increased sensitivity to NDPs in newborn and young infants, and dose requirements are reduced during anaesthesia with inhalational agents. Variation between individual patients is high.[38] Thus small doses should be given first and the effect noted. The influence of the inhalational agents on the clinical effect of NDPs is profound and should always be taken into account.[39]

d-*Tubocurarine and pancuronium*

d-Tubocurarine and pancuronium can appropriately be called 'long-acting relaxants' since a single 'intubating' dose (500 μg kg^{-1} of tubocurarine or 150 μg kg^{-1} pancuronium) will provide relaxation for up to 1 h, especially in the presence of inhalational agents.

d-Tubocurarine will cause a predictable fall in blood pressure, associated with the release of histamine. Pancuronium (100 μg kg^{-1}) provides useful relaxation for about 45 min. It is still widely used in paediatric practice, particularly for cardiac surgery where its vagolytic properties can be used to good effect in opposing the bradycardia engendered by large doses of fentanyl. Many anaesthetists have now abandoned these older agents in shorter surgical procedures in an attempt to minimize difficulties with reversal at the termination of surgery. In intensive care, the use of bolus doses of long-acting relaxants is gradually being superseded by infusions of the shorter-acting atracurium or vecuronium.

The advent of the shorter-acting NDPs atracurium and vecuronium has made it possible to use minimal amounts of the agent to obtain a desired effect. Bolus doses are suitable for procedures of say, up to one hour, an infusion (monitored with a peripheral nerve stimulator) being used if the procedure is more prolonged. Both these drugs are easy to reverse even after prolonged administration and significant cumulation does not occur. For these reasons the longer acting agents *d*-tubocurarine and pancuronium can be avoided in routine paediatric practice.

Atracurium

The kinetics of this drug have been well studied in paediatric patients. Most of the dose is cleared by liver esterases. The remainder is metabolized by non-specific plasma esterases or undergoes spontaneous hydrolysis in the plasma. In both children and adults, ester hydrolysis to a quaternary acid or alcohol with further degradation to laudanosine is the main pathway of elimination. Only a small amount of the breakdown occurs via spontaneous hydrolysis (Hofmann biotransformation) which produces initially laudanosine and a laudanosine-quaternary monoacrylate component. This is further broken down to laudanosine and the residual acrylate bridge. Laudanosine is known to be a potent CNS stimulant in animal models but the clinical significance of this is not yet evaluated. There are no reports of toxicity in humans after clinical use of atracurium although cumulation of laudanosine may cause an increase in anaesthetic requirements. Pseudocholinesterase deficiency has no significant effect, non-specific esterases being largely involved. Atracurium does not cause significant release of histamine in children.[40]

On a surface area basis, the ED_{95} of atracurium in infants is lower than that in older children.[41,42] Kinetic data shows alpha and beta half-lives which differ considerably between infants and older children.[43] The distribution volume is larger and the elimination half-life shorter in infants under two years than in either older children or adults. Bolus doses of 500 μg kg^{-1} are usually used followed by infusion of 500 μg kg^{-1} h^{-1} or boluses according to the response to the peripheral nerve stimulator.

Vecuronium

Vecuronium has a steroidal molecule similar to that of pancuronium. It is excreted unchanged in the bile to the extent of 50–70 per cent and by the kidney (up to 15 per cent). Limited metabolism occurs; potential metabolites are 3-hydroxy-, 17-hydroxy-, and 3,17-dihydroxy vecuronium. 3-hydroxy vecuronium is pharmacologically active at the neuromuscular junction.

Dosage requirements are higher for children than in infants or adults.[44,45] In infants, a large dose ($2 \times ED_{95}$) produces a duration of clinical effect *twice* as long as that seen in older children. Thus, neuromuscular blockade is best monitored with a nerve stimulator.

As with atracurium the volume of distribution is larger in infants[46] than older children but clearance (unlike atracurium) is similar in both groups. Bolus doses of 100 μg kg^{-1} of vecuronium are usually given followed by infusion of up to 100 μg kg^{-1} h^{-1} or boluses of 50–100 μg kg^{-1} according to the response to nerve stimulation.

Mivacurium

Mivacurium is a short-acting muscle relaxant recently introduced to the UK market. It is a benzyloquinonium compound composed of 3 stereoisomers (cis-cis, cis-trans and trans-trans). Cis-trans and trans-trans have very high clearances and small volumes of distribution resulting in the short elimination half-life of two minutes. The cis-cis isomer is longer-acting but only constitutes 4–8 per cent of the total drug. Dose requirement is higher in children than in adults; good intubating conditions are provided by 150 μg kg^{-1} especially when the block is potentiated by volatile agents.[47] The ED_{95} in children aged 2–12 years is 100 μg kg^{-1}. It has a faster onset, shorter duration of block and faster spontaneous recovery in this age group compared with adults.[48] 100 μg kg^{-1} provides clinically acceptable relaxation for about 7 minutes and 200 μg kg^{-1} for 10 minutes. Children require more frequent doses than adults to maintain the block, further increments of 100 μg kg^{-1} producing continued neuromuscular blockade for about 7 minutes. Infusion rates for 95 per cent block in infants in one study was 820 (SD 300), μg kg^{-1} h^{-1}, a figure similar to that quoted for children during balanced narcotic anaesthesia.[49] Spontaneous recovery after a dose of mivacurium is complete in 10 minutes. The main metabolic pathway is hydrolysis by plasma cholinesterase to a quaternary alcohol and a quaternary ester, which are clinically inactive. The block is not prolonged unless plasma cholinesterase activity is less than 20 per cent of normal. Hydrolysis also occurs in the liver and small amounts are eliminated in bile and urine.[50]

Cardiovascular effects are generally insignificant with mild flushing, hypotension, and tachycardia occasionally occurring. Mivacurium has no vagolytic or ganglion-blocking properties. Urticaria and bronchospasm are reported but rare and one case of asystole has been recently cited in the literature.[51]

Rocuronium

The aminosteroid rocuronium (ORG 9426) is an analogue of vecuronium but with a more rapid onset of action (about twice as rapid as vecuronium).

Its duration of action is similar to that of vecuronium. Slightly higher doses (ED_{50}, ED_{90}, and ED_{95}) are required for infants than adults during halothane anaesthesia. 500 μg kg^{-1} produces 95–100 per cent block. The duration of action reported by Motsch et al.[52] is about 15 minutes in children, less than that reported in adults, and is comparable to vecuronium in children aged 1–4 years. Only minor effects on blood pressure were noted, there were moderate increases in heart rate (approximately 20 beats min^{-1} in children aged 1–4 years and 10 beats min^{-1} in older children aged 5–10 years). No clinical effects attributable to histamine release have been reported.

Side-effects

With all competitive neuromuscular blocking drugs the unwanted effects after an appropriate dose are mainly on the cardiovascular system (although bronchospasm may occur following histamine release). The effect may be mediated by histamine, ganglion blockade, or vagal blockade. Furthermore, the polypharmaceutical nature of anaesthesia may result in liberation of histamine by several drugs. In adults d-tubocurarine releases more histamine than atracurium, although the effect of atracurium is minimal in infants and children.[53] Vecuronium does not cause liberation of histamine.

Pancuronium is well known to have a vagolytic effect, thereby increasing the heart rate. This effect has proved useful in counteracting the bradycardia produced, for example, by larger doses of fentanyl. Bradycardia may occur when either vecuronium rocuronium, or atracurium are used with fentanyl (or alfentanil) without an anticholinergic agent.

Reversal of neuromuscular blockade

Although the advent of shorter-acting agents and the use of infusions have reduced the necessity for pharmacological reversal in many patients, it is the authors' view that reversal should be undertaken in all neonates and infants, especially if long-acting agents such as d-tubocurarine or pancuronium have been used. Reversal agents should be given only after spontaneous recovery has started to occur as shown by the response to the peripheral nerve stimulator. Doses up to 50 μg kg^{-1} of neostigmine with an anticholinergic drug such as atropine 20 μg kg^{-1} or glycopyrronium 10 μg kg^{-1} may be required to restore full muscle power as judged by the ability to lift the head to the same extent as pre-operatively. Edrophonium has been used but in the doses normally employed has not been shown to offer any significant advantages clinically. In large doses, however, it is longer lasting with fewer side-effects. Monitoring of neuromuscular function is desirable to enable minimal amounts of relaxants to be used while ensuring full clinical effect. Non-depolarizing muscle relaxants are potentiated by inhalational agents, aminoglycoside antibiotics, hypothermia, reduced muscle blood flow, acidosis, and hypocalcaemia. Little or no relaxant is required in myasthenia. Such interactions may complicate reversal at the end of the procedure, the child failing to breathe despite commonly used doses of neostigmine.

OPIOIDS AND OTHER ANALGESICS

Opium has been used in medicine for thousands of years and the most active ingredient, morphine, or drugs that act in the same way, are still the most useful and most widely applicable pain relieving agents. *Opioid* (lit: like opium) is the term used for agents which bind to opioid receptors[54,55] and opioid receptors are those which bind to the morphine antagonist naloxone.

There are three kinds of opioid receptor: mu (μ), delta (δ), and kappa (κ) which act on the pre- and post-synaptic membranes of nociceptor afferent neurones.

Mu and delta agonists have an effect in three ways: by enhancing potassium efflux, thereby hyperpolarizing the membrane; either directly or mediated through a regulatory inhibitory G-protein which also reduces the formation of cyclic AMP and indirectly on calcium influx and intracellular calcium levels. Alpha-2 sympathomimetic agonists such as clonidine, gamma-aminobutyric acid at the B receptor (and other agents) act in the same way. Tolerance to these drugs, at least in the short term, is by uncoupling of the receptor–effector protein complex, rather than by reduction of the number of receptors. Sigma (σ) receptors are not bound by naloxone and are not classed as opioid; activity is mainly excitatory (mydriasis, increased heart rate, increased ventilation, and hallucinations). σ agonists are often the less active optical isomer of opioids which are used as antitussives (e.g. dextrorphan, dextromethorphan). They can be effective against secondary neurogenic pain either by binding to the sigma receptor or by their cross selectivity with the NMDA receptor.

Mu and delta receptor activation causes insensitivity by hyperpolarization mainly by increasing potassium efflux. Kappa receptor activation reduces nociception largely by altering calcium flux, but kappa agonists are effective against fewer kinds of pain than mu and delta agonists. All three actions can potentiate each other and the simultaneous release of the endogenous morphine-like substances *endorphins* — beta-endorphin, (mu and delta) enkephalin (mainly delta, some mu), and dynorphin (mainly kappa) — in times of injury or excitement can produce powerful inhibition of pain. Predominantly delta receptor agonists are not yet available, but methadone, with significant delta-agonist activity, may be useful in children who have become tolerant to mu agonists because of intrapartum or postpartum exposure to the drugs.

Endorphin levels are high immediately after birth and opioid receptors are present more densely than in the adult. Inactivation of some of the opioid receptors and reduction in their number occurs in the weeks and months following birth. This may account for the relative lack of obvious distress in neonates during stressful or painful procedures. Opioids are effective in most forms of pain, nocigenic and inflammatory, visceral and parietal, but, because the receptors are present at synapses, they are more effective in pain which is served by multi-synaptic C-fibre spinoreticular pathways, than the sharp pain such as pin prick which is traditionally associated with the A δ fibres and few synapses of the spinothalamic pathway. The sharp pain of cough or sneeze in the presence of an abdominal wound is better prevented by afferent nerve blockade.

Side-effects

Opioid receptors are present throughout the brain and spinal cord and in many other organs. Their actions at sites other than the nociceptive pathways limit their use. The respiratory neurones of the pons and medulla are associated with opioid receptors and opioids decrease the sensitivity of these neurones to carbon dioxide and also alter the rhythm of ventilation to include longer periods of apnoea. Total ventilation is decreased with the rate reduced relatively more than the tidal volume. Gut motility is depressed and the secretions of the gut are reduced. Opioids indirectly stimulate the chemoreceptor trigger zone and the vomiting centre of the area postrema in the floor of the fourth ventricle and cause nausea and vomiting. They cause itch, especially when applied epidurally or intrathecally.

Clinical use of opioids

Many paediatric anaesthetists have hitherto been wary of employing opioids in anaesthetic techniques for small babies. This is largely based on the knowledge that postoperative apnoea is very likely, especially in the premature infant. However, apnoea may occur following any anaesthetic, even if no opioids are used, and is said to be common in premature babies up to 60 weeks post-conceptual age.[56]

Opioids have, however, been successfully employed in neonatal anaesthesia without postoperative ventilation. Postoperative apnoea monitoring is mandatory in all neonates.

Morphine

Morphine is relatively lipid-insoluble (methadone is 82 times, diamorphine 200 times, fentanyl 580 times, and sufentanil 1270 times more soluble in lipid than morphine). Morphine is poorly distributed beyond the blood–brain barrier in the adult. Similarly, offset of clinical action is delayed after the fall of the plasma concentration below that required for the onset of that action. Elimination is mainly by conjugation with both glucuronide and sulphate[57] in the neonate and most is eliminated in the urine. Some is excreted through the bile to the gut from which bacterial breakdown of the conjugate allows reabsorption back into the plasma. In renal failure, significant amounts of morphine 6-glucuronide accumulate and this metabolite is both more polar and more potent than morphine. Elimination half-life is approximately twice as long in the neonate as in the adult (see Table 2.3) and morphine should be used only in those clinical areas in which it is possible to assist ventilation.

In addition to those side-effects mentioned above, morphine may cause hypotension possibly because of histamine release. It has little effect on cardiac output although myocardial oxygen consumption and left ventricular end-diastolic pressure may be decreased. Because the volume of distribution at steady state is relatively small and the offset of effect is dependent more on elimination, morphine is more suitable for use by infusion than are the more lipid soluble opioids such as fentanyl or sufentanil.

Pethidine

Pethidine is more soluble than morphine, faster acting but less potent and effective. It has two major metabolites: norpethidine and pethidinic acid and their conjugates. Norpethidine has excitatory properties and may cause hypertension, hyperthermia, and convulsions.[58] Accumulation of this metabolite is more likely to occur with repeated doses and with depression of

Table 2.3 Pharmacokinetics of morphine — variation with age

Age	Clearance $(ml.kg^{-1}min^{-1})$	β half-life (hours)
1–7 days	5.5	7.2
1–3 months	10.5	6.2
3–6 months	13.9	4.5
6 months–2.5 years	21.7	2.3
Adults	23.0	1.7

Adapted from Table 2.2 in "Neonatal anaesthetic pharmacology" by G. Meakin in *A Handbook of Neonatal Anaesthesia* (Ed Hughes D.G., Mather S.J., and Wolf A.R.). WB Saunders Co London (1995) p. 30.

the oxidase metabolic pathway or when large doses are required because of congenital or acquired tolerance to opioids. As with most other opioids, the elimination half-life is greater in neonates than in adults.

Fentanyl

High dose fentanyl has been employed routinely in cardiac anaesthesia for some years but recently interest has developed in the use of opioids for shorter procedures in general paediatric surgery. One study[59] has highlighted the hormonal response which neonates are able to mount to stress and its amelioration by fentanyl. In small (1 μg kg^{-1}) doses, fentanyl has little effect on cardiac output or blood pressure. Higher doses may lead to bradycardia and a fall in blood pressure unless an anticholinergic drug is also given. Chest wall rigidity necessitating muscle relaxation may also occur with high doses. Full term neonates have a clearance for fentanyl which is similar to that in the older child or adult but it is reduced in the premature neonate. Various studies report differing elimination half-lives in neonates but it appears to be significantly prolonged by comparison with adults. Post-operative respiratory depression for several hours is a possibility after repeated doses or infusions.

Alfentanil

Alfentanil is a potent analgesic which is distinguished by having a very rapid onset and the shortest duration of any of the opioids in current use. It is about one-quarter as potent as fentanyl on a weight basis. Unlike fentanyl the short duration of effect is still seen after multiple doses and cumulation is minimal. There is little effect on cardiac output or peripheral resistance. The drug is rapidly metabolized to inactive metabolites. Alfentanil is being used clinically in neonatal anaesthesia and is popular in paediatric anaesthesia in general. Its short elimination half-life[60] (about 60 min in children and 90 min in adults) makes it suitable for use by infusion (loading dose 15–20 μg kg^{-1} followed by 1 μg kg^{-1} min^{-1}). Very little has yet been published with regard to the pharmacokinetics in small children.

Sufentanil

Sufentanil is now becoming popular for long procedures. It is six or seven times more potent than fentanyl but bradycardia is less likely to occur. The hormonal stress response is well obtunded with doses of 15 μg kg^{-1}.[61] Sequential studies with sufentanil during the first week of life and at subsequent operations between 3 and 4 weeks of age in patients with cardiovascular disease showed maturation of sufentanil metabolism as revealed by increased clearance and elimination half-life.[62] Elimination half-life is similar to infants and children at about 50 min, about one third of the adult value. Clearance is 30 per cent higher than in adults.

Phenoperidine

Phenoperidine causes profound respiratory depression and falls in blood pressure but also gives good operative conditions. It is only occasionally used in paediatric anaesthesia.

Remifentanil

This is a new mu opioid currently in development. It has a potency similar to fentanyl but is extremely short-acting being metabolized by non-specific esterases and having a half-life of less than ten minutes. It has an active metabolite which is one-thousand times less potent than remifentanil. The half-life is almost context-insensitive, that is the half-life is the same after a prolonged infusion as after a brief one, and the same after a large dose as after a small one. It is reversed by naloxone, but the speed of reversal is matched by the effect of discontinuation of the infusion. Because of its short action it can be used in large doses to reduce stress or allow smaller doses of general anaesthetic agents to be given. However, it can cause rigidity of truncal or laryngeal muscles, and muscle relaxation and ventilation may be required.

Partial and weak agonist opioids

Some opioids possess agonist properties at opioid receptors while having an inherent antagonist activity which limits analgesia and respiratory depression even when repeated doses are given. They can also be used in a sequential technique to allow reversal of a potent agonist drug in the recovery period without sacrificing analgesia.

A weak agonist (e.g. codeine) may be capable of achieving a powerful effect but in high doses: it has a low potency. A strong, full agonist is capable of achieving a powerful effect in relatively low doses and by occupying relatively few of the available receptors. Increasing the dose achieves an increasing effect. A partial agonist (e.g. buprenorphine) achieves a clinically significant effect by occupying a large proportion of the available receptors, and maximal effect is less than that of a full agonist. However, unless the affinity to the receptors is poor, this receptor binding denies some receptors to another agonist or to endogenous opioid substances. It can therefore act as an antagonist. A drug such as naloxone, which has a high receptor affinity but no noticeable intrinsic effect, is called a full antagonist.

A drug can be a partial agonist at one receptor, a full agonist at another, and an antagonist at a third. The action of a mixed and/or partial agonist therefore depends upon the relative affinities and intrinsic activities at each receptor, the saturation of each receptor, and the synergism or antagonism of other drugs. The relative affinities of some common 'partial' agonists are listed in Table 2.4. Interaction between full and partial agonists can be complex. If the partial agonist and the full agonist are present in low concentration and each occupies a small proportion of the total number of receptors the effect is additive. If the partial agonist is present in high concentration and occupies a large proportion or all of the receptors and has a high affinity for these receptors, the receptors are denied to a full agonist and the action of the full agonist is blocked or antagonized. If most of the receptors are occupied by a full agonist, and a partial agonist with a high affinity for the receptor is introduced, the effect of the full agonist will be reduced.

Buprenorphine has a long duration of action and can be given sublingually. However, sublingual administration is not as effective as the intramuscular or intravenous route; the peak levels are reduced and the action is less prolonged. One study found buprenorphine given sublingually to be equivalent in duration to intramuscular morphine in children but longer when both drugs were given intravenously.[63] Buprenorphine has a greater affinity for the μ receptor than naloxone, and ventilatory depression caused by buprenorphine is more difficult to reverse by this means. Many agonist/antagonist drugs produce dysphoria, presumably by action on sigma receptors.

Nalbuphine is a kappa agonist with only a weak action at the sigma receptor. Nalbuphine causes fewer hallucinations or dysphoric symptoms than pentazocine or butorphanol but the somnolence it causes may sometimes be associated with vivid unpleasant dreams rather than sedation. Despite its relatively safe agonist profile, ventilatory depression can still be produced. It is about one third as potent as morphine for body-wall pain, it produces less cardiovascular changes than morphine, and has a lower incidence of nausea.[64]

Table 2.4 Receptor selectivity of partial agonist opioid analgesics

Drug	Receptor type			
	μ	κ	δ	σ
Pentazocine	pA	A	ant	A
Butorphanol	pA	A	Ant	A
Nalbuphine	Ant	pA	ant	a
Buprenorphine	pA	Ant	A	

A, strong agonist; pA, partial agonist; Ant, strong antagonist; ant, weak antagonist; a, weak agonist
Reproduced from Alexander and Hill (1987). *Postoperative pain control*. Blackwell Scientific Publications, Oxford.

Naloxone

Naloxone is a potent antagonist at the μ and δ receptors but less potent at the κ receptor.

It reverses the ventilatory depressant effect of the μ receptor opioid agonists but reverses less completely κ agonists such as pentazocine or high-affinity receptor binders such as buprenorphine.

It can also displace endogenous opioids from their receptor sites, increasing stress which may be harmful.[65] Small doses of 1–2 μg kg^{-1} should be titrated against the effect. It has a shorter action than most commonly used opioid analgesics and repeated doses or an infusion may be required to antagonise unwanted opioid effects. (Doses and an infusion table are given in the appendix, see p. 272.)

Clonidine

The opioids act as analgesics either very powerfully within the brain or, less powerfully within the spinal cord. Opioid binding within the mid-brain stimulates other descending pathways which release either noradrenaline or serotonin (5-hydroxytryptamine) within the dorsal horn of the spinal cord. Noradrenaline acts on the alpha-2 adrenergic receptors to produce analgesia.

Clonidine is an incompletely selective alpha-2 agonist, mimicking the action of noradrenaline at this receptor. Presynaptically, it acts to inhibit the release of noradrenaline, thereby causing hypotension and somnolence. It also inhibits the release of substance P. Pre- and post-synaptically, it acts like a μ opioid agonist to hyperpolarize neuronal membranes to inhibit nociceptive impulses, but acts on different receptors. Clonidine can therefore reduce the required concentration of other anaesthetic agents for surgery and potentiates the action of opioids, especially when applied epidurally or intrathecally.

Tramadol

This is an analgesic which has been in use in Germany for nearly two decades but has only recently sought a wider market. It has several actions which potentiate each other. It is a very week mu opioid, approximately two thousand times less potent than morphine. It also increases the availability of both serotonin and noradrenaline within the spinal cord. The combined potentiation of these actions yields an agent which is less effective than pethidine but more than codeine in the recommended doses. The action of ventilatory depression or gut motility depression is extremely small, but the incidence of nausea is similar and that of sweating slightly greater than that of most opioids.

Non-steroidal anti-inflammatory drugs (NSAIDs) and paracetamol

These drugs inhibit the formation of prostaglandins, NSAIDs principally in the peripheral tissue and paracetamol almost entirely within the brain. They are antipyretic and NSAIDs are anti-inflammatory.

Prostaglandin inhibits the calcium-activated prolonged potassium efflux and post-potential hyperpolarization of the C-fibre nociceptor or neurone, thereby allowing the faster generation of impulses and more stimulation of the pain centres. The lack of correlation between anti-inflammatory activity in post-inflammation analgesia or between prostaglandin-inhibiting activity and either anti-inflammatory or analgesic activity indicates efficacy by other mechanisms. These include differential inhibition of the different prosta-glandin synthase isoenzymes, differential penetration into inflamed tissues or brain, descending serotonergic activation and interaction with nitric oxide and the NMDA and non-NMDA glutamate receptors, and other actions on arachidonic acid and phospholipase.

These drugs are effective for mild to moderate pain, especially inflamma-tory type pain or pain resulting from the action of prostaglandin such as spasm of the bowel, bile duct, urethra, or fallopian tubes.

The inhibition of prostaglandin synthesis also limits the use of NSAIDs because prostaglandins are required to maintain the healing processes of the gut lining, to limit the effect of acid in the stomach, to increase renal blood flow when this is reduced below normal, to promote laminar blood flow, and maintain the normal sequence of clotting. NSAIDS therefore have greater risks in the presence of gastric damage or ulceration, in hypovolaemia, heart failure, or when used at the same time as cyclosporin, or when bleeding from fractures, thoraco-abdominal wounds, or tonsil beds is likely to be large and unnoticed or uncorrected. NSAIDs are also contraindicated in adults with asthma because of the small proportion in whom bronchospasm can be made worse, although NSAIDs are freely used in asthmatic children by many prac-titioners as NSAID-induced asthma seems to be very rare in younger children.

Although several NSAIDs have been licensed for use in arthritis in chil-dren, at present only ibuprofen has a licence for postoperative pain in chil-dren (over 7 kg, approximately 1 year of age). Other NSAIDs are, however widely used in children, particularly diclofenac, which is often given rectally for postoperative pain.

REFERENCES

1. Cook, D. R. (1974). Neonatal anaesthetic pharmacology: a review. *Anesthesia and Analgesia*, **53**, 544.
2. Cook, D. R. (1976). Pediatric anaesthesia: pharmacological considerations. *Drugs*, **12**, 212.

3. Friss-Hansen, B. (1971). Body composition during growth. *Pediatrics*, **47**, 264.
4. Guignard, J. P. *et al.* (1975). Glomerular filtration during the first 3 weeks of life. *Journal of Pedatrics*, **87**, 268.
5. Stoelting, R. K. and Longnecker, D. E. (1972). Effect of right to left shunt on rate of increase in arterial anaesthetic concentration. *Anesthesiology*, **36**, 352.
6. Lerman, J. *et al.* (1984). Age and solubility of volatile anaesthetics in blood. *Anesthesiology*, **61**, 139.
7. Solanitre, E. and Rackow, H. (1969). The pulmonary exchange of nitrous oxide and halothane in infants and children. *Anesthesiology*, **30**, 388.
8. Brandom, B. W., Brandom, R. B., and Cook, D. R. (1983). Uptake and distribution of halothane in infants: in vitro measurements and computer simulations. *Anesthesia and Analgesia*, **62**, 404.
9. Oldendorf, W. H. *et al.* (1972). Blood brain barrier: penetration of morphine codeine, heroin and methadone after carotid injection. *Science*, **178**, 984.
10. Bayon, A. *et al.* Perinatal development of the endorphin and enkephalin containing systems in rat brain. *Brain Research*, **179**, 93.
11. Lerman, J. *et al.* (1983). Anaesthetic requirements for halothane in young children 0–1 month and 1–6 months of age. *Anesthesiology*, **59**, 421.
12. Gregory, G. A. *et al.* (1983). Fetal anaesthetic requirement (MAC) for halothane. *Anesthesia and Analgesia*, **62**, 9.
13. Cooke, D. R. *et al.* (1981). The inspired median effective dose, brain concentration at anesthesia and cardiovascular index for halothane in young rats. *Anesthesia and Analgesia*, **60**, 182.
14. Hickey, P. R. *et al.* (1986). Pulmonary and systemic haemodynamic effects of nitrous oxide in infants with normal and elevated pulmonary vascular resistance. *Anesthesiology*, **65**, 374.
15. Fisher, D. E. *et al.* (1984). Comparison of enflurane, halothane and isoflurane for outpatient pediatric anesthesia. *Anesthesiology*, **61A**, 427.
16. Frink, B. J. Junior, Malan, T. P., Atlas, M. *et al.* (1992). Clinical comparison of sevoflurane and isoflurane in healthy patients. *Anesthesia and Analgesia*, **74**, 241.
17. Ghouri, A. F., Bodner, M., and White, P. F. (1991). Recovery profile after desflurane–nitrous oxide v isoflurane–nitrous oxide in outpatients. *Anesthesiology*, **74**, 419.
18. Black, G. W., Hatch, D. J., and Morris, P. (1987). Halothane hepatitis in children. *British Medical Journal*, **285**, 117.
19. Wark, H. *et al.* (1990). Halothane metabolism in children. *British Journal of Anaesthesia*, **64**, 474.
20. Neal, M. B. *et al.* (1984). Haemodynamic and cardiovascular effects of halothane and isoflurane anesthesia in children. *Anesthesiology*, **61A**, 437.
21. Barash, P. G. *et al.* (1978). Ventricular function in children during halothane anesthesia: an echocardiographic evaluation. *Anesthesiology*, **49**, 79.
22. Gregory, G. A. (1982). The baroresponses of preterm infants during halothane anaesthesia. *Canadian Anaesthetists' Society Journal*, $29, 105
23. Bjorkman, S. *et al.* (1987). Pharmacokinetics of IV and rectal methohexitone in children. *British Journal of Anesthesia*, **59**, 1541.
24. Grant, I. S. and Mackenzie, N. (1985). Recovery following propofol anaesthesia — a review of 3 different anaesthetic techniques. *Postgraduate Medical Journal*, **61** (Suppl. 3), 129.
25. Hanallah, R. *et al.* (1990). Induction dose of propofol in unpremedicated children. *Anesthesia and Analgesia*, **70**, Suppl. 143.

26. Sharples, A., Shaw, E. A., and Meakin, G. (1994). Recovery times following induction of anaesthesia with propofol, methohexitone, enflurane or thiopentone in children. *Paediatric Anaesthesia*, **4**, 101.

27. Scott, R. P. F., Saunders, D. A., and Norman, J. (1988). Propofol: clinical strategies for preventing the pain of injection. *Anaesthesia*, **43**, 492.

28. Thompson, K. (1994). Experience with midazolam as a paediatric medication on board ship. *Today's Anaesthetist*, **9**, 142.

29. Karl,, W., Keifer A. T., Rosenberger, J. L., Larach, M. G., and Ruffle, J. M. (1992). Comparison of the safety and efficacy of intranasal midazolam or sufentanil for preinduction of anesthesia in pediatric patients. *Anesthesiology*, **76**, 209.

30. McCluskey, A. and Meakin, G. H. (1994). Oral administration of midazolam as a premedicant for paediatric day case anaesthesia. *Anaesthesia*, **49**, 782.

31. Goudsouzian, N. G. (1980). Maturation of neuromuscular transmission in the infant. *British Journal of Anaesthesia*, **52**, 205.

32. Cook, D. R. and Fischer, C. G. (1975). Neuromuscular blocking effects of succinylcholine in infants and children. *Anesthesiology*, **42**, 662.

33. Walts, L. F. and Dillon, J. B. (1969). The response of newborns to succinylcholine and d-tubocurarine. *Anesthesiology*, **31**, 35.

34. Goudsouzian, N. G. and Liu, L. M. P. (1984). The neuromuscular response of infants to a continuous infusion of succinylcholine. *Anesthesiology*, **60**, 97.

35. Goudsouzian, N. G., Liu, L. M. P., and Cote, C. J. (1981). Comparison of equipotent doses of non-depolarizing muscle relaxants in children. *Anesthesia and Analgesia*, **60**, 862.

36. Goudsouzian, N. G., Ryan, J. F., and Savarese, J. J. (1974). The neuromuscular effects of pancuronium in infants and children. *Anesthesiology*, **41**, 95.

37. Goudsouzian, N. G., Martyn, J. J. A., and Liu, L. M. P. (1984). The dose-response effect of long-acting non-depolarizing neuromuscular blocking agents in children. *Canadian Anaesthetists' Society Journal*, **3**, 246.

38. Goudsouzian, N. G. *et al.* (1975). Re-evaluation of dosage and duration of action of d-tubocurarine in the paediatric age group. *Anesthesiology*, **43**, 416.

39. Brandom, B. W., Rudd, G. D., and Cook, D. R. (1983). Clinical pharmacology of atracurium in paediatric patients. *British Journal of Anaesthesia*, **55** (Suppl.), 117.

40. Stiller, R. L., Cook, D. R., and Chakravorti, S. (1985). In vitro degradation of atracurium in human plasma. *British Journal of Anaesthesia*, **57**, 1085.

41. Caruso, P. and Moszczynski, B. S. (1988). Histamine release after atracurium in children. *Anesthesiology*, **69**, (Suppl. A), 762.

42. Brandom, B. W. *et al.* (1984). Clinical pharmacology of atracurium in infants. *Anesthesia and Analgesia*, **63**, 309.

43. Brandom, B. W. *et al.* (1986). Pharmacokinetics of atracurium in infants and children. *British Journal of Anaesthesia*, **58**, 1210.

44. Meretoja, O. A., Wirtavuori, K., and Neuvonen, P. J. (1988). Age dependence of the dose-response curve of vecuronium in paediatric patients during balanced anesthesia. *Anesthesia and Analgesia*, **67**, 21.

45. Schippers, H. C. *et al.* (1988). Dose-response curve of vecuronium bromide in anesthetised neonates, infants and children. *Anesthesiology*, **69** (Suppl. A), 761.

46. Fisher, D. M. (1985). Pharmacodynamics of vecuronium in infants and children. *Clinical Pharmacology and Therapeutics*, **37**, 402.

47. Sarner, J. B., Brandom, B. W., Woelfel, S. K. *et al.* (1989). Clinical pharmacology of mivacurium chloride (BW 109OU) in children during nitrous oxide-halothane and nitrous oxide-narcotic anesthesia. *Anesthesia and Analgesia*, **68**, 116.

48. Goudsouzian, N. G., Alifimoff, J. K., Eberley, C. *et al.* (1989). Neuromuscular and cardiovascular effects of mivacurium in children. *Anesthesiology*, **70**, 237.
49. Brandom, B. W., Sarner, J. E. B., Woelfel, S. K. *et al.* (1990). Mivacurium infusion requirement in pediatric surgical patients during nitrous oxide-halothane and during nitrous oxide-narcotic anesthesia. *Anesthesia and Analgesia*, **71**, 16.
50. Meretoja, O. A., Taivainen, T., and Wirtavuori, K. (1994). Pharmacodynamics of mivacurium in infants. *British Journal of Anaesthesia*, **73**, 490.
51. Else, T. A. (1994). Asystole associated with mivacurium (letter). *Anaesthesia*, **49**, 926.
52. Motsch, J., Leuwer, M., Pfau, M. *et al.* (1994). Time course of action and recovery of rocuronium bromide in children during halothane anaesthesia — a preliminary report. *European Journal of Anaesthesiology*, **11** (59), 75.
53. Brandom, B. W. *et al.* (1984). Clinical pharmacology of atracurium in infants. *Anesthesia and Analgesia*, **63**, 309.
54. Pert, C. B. and Snyder, D. H. (1973). Opiate receptor: demonstration in nervous tissue. *Science*, **179**, 1011.
54. Simon, E. J., Hiller, J. M., and Edelman, I. (1973). Stereo-specific binding of the potent narcotic ^{3}H-etorphine to cat brain homogenate. *Proceedings of the National Academy of Sciences USA*, **70**, 1947.
56. Kurth, C. D. *et al.* (1987). Postoperative apnea in preterm infants. *Anesthesiology*, **66**, 483.
57. Lynn, A. M. and Slattery, J. T. (1987). Morphine pharmacokinetics in early infancy. *Anesthesiology*, **66**, 136.
58. Szeto, H. H. and Intureisi, C. E. (1976). Simultaneous determination of meperidine and normeperidine in biofluids. *Journal of Chromatography*, **125**, 503.
59. Anand, K. J. S., Sippell, W. G., and Aynsley-Green, A. (1987). Randomized trial of fentanyl anaesthesia in preterm babies undergoing surgery. *Lancet*, **I**, 243.
60. Roure, P. *et al.* (1987). Pharmacokinetics of alfentanil in children undergoing surgery. *British Journal of Anaesthesia*, **59**, 1437.
61. Davis, P. J. *et al.* (1987). Pharmacodynamics and pharmacokinetics of high dose sufentanil in infants and children. *Anesthesia and Analgesia*, **66**, 203.
62. Greely, W. J. and de Bruijn, N. P. (1988). Changes in sufentanil pharmacokinetics within the neonatal period. *Anesthesia and Analgesia*, **67**, 86.
63. Maunuksela, E. L., Korpela, R., and Olkkou, K. T. (1988). Comparison of buprenorphine with morphine in the treatment of post-operative pain in children. *Anesthesia and Analgesia*, **67**, 233.
64. Hughes, D. G. (1988). Nalbuphine for post-operative pain relief in children. *Schmerz/Pain/Douleur*, **9**, 52.
65. Peters, W. P. *et al.* (1981). Pressor effect of naloxone in septic shock. *Lancet*, **I**, 529.

FURTHER READING

Muto, R. *et al.* (1993). Initial experience of complete switchover to sevoflurane in 1550 children. *Paediatric Anaesthesia*, **3**, 229.
Mannion, D., Casey, W., and Doherty, P. (1994). Desflurane in paediatric anaesthesia. *Paediatric Anaesthesia*, **4**, 301.

Jones, R. D. M., Chan, K., and Andrew, L. J. (1990). Pharmacokinetics of propofol in children. *British Journal of Anaesthesia*, **65**, 661.

Anderson, G. *et al.* (1994). Rectal midazolam as premedicant in children: a dose-response study. *Paediatric Anaesthesia*, **4**, 365.

Meakin, G., Walker, R. W. M., and Dearlove, O. R. (1990) Myotonic and neuro-muscular blocking effects of increased doses of suxamethonium in infants and children. *British Journal of Anaesthesia*, **65**, 816.

Fisher, D. M. *et al.* (1990). Pharmacokinetics and pharmacodynamics of atracurium in infants and children. *Anesthesiology*, **73**, 33.

Brahen, N. H. *et al.* (1990). Plasma sufentanil levels in paediatric outpatients receiving nasal pre-induction of anaesthesia. *Anesthesia and Analgesia*, **70**, Suppl. 33.

Baptista, J. S. and Dias, M. C. (1993). Post-operative analgesia with caudal epidural sufentanil. *Paediatric Anaesthesia*, **3**, 371.

Tobias, J. D. and Rasmussen, G. E. (1995). Transnasal butorphanol for postoperative analgesia following paediatric surgery in a third-world country. *Paediatric Anaesthesia*, **5**, 63.

Lönnqvist, P. A. and Bergendahl, H. (1993). Pharmacokinetics and haemodynamic response after an intravenous bolus injection of clonidine in children. *Paediatric Anaesthesia*, **3**, 359.

3

Paediatric anaesthetic apparatus

D. G. Hughes

BREATHING SYSTEMS

The T-piece

The most commonly used paediatric breathing system in the UK is the modified Ayre's T-piece. This system was introduced by Philip Ayre in 1937.[1] In his anaesthetic practice for neurosurgery and plastic surgery he found it difficult to prevent hypoxaemia with his existing apparatus and so designed a circuit to eliminate both this and rebreathing. This consisted of a metal T-piece of 1 cm internal diameter connected to an endotracheal tube by a short piece of rubber tubing. The anaesthetic gases were delivered through the narrow limb of the T-piece and the other limb remained open for air entrainment.

In 1950, Jackson Rees modified this circuit initially by attaching a short expiratory limb which then avoided the problem of air entrainment as long as its volume exceeded the infant's tidal volume. By using an open tailed 500 ml reservoir bag on the end of this expiratory limb, Jackson Rees enabled spontaneous ventilation to be monitored more safely. It also allowed ventilation by hand and later by appropriately designed paediatric ventilators. The original T-piece has been considerably modified over the years.[2]

The Jackson Rees modification is classified as Mapleson Type E (see Fig. 3.1.). Since its first introduction the T-piece has been altered to allow for factors which are important in small infants. These are:

- dead space;
- resistance;
- humidity;
- bulk of the equipment.

1. *Minimal dead space.* An increase in dead space of a few ml will dramatically reduce the alveolar ventilation of a full-term neonate, and even more so in a premature infant (see Table 3.1.).

2. *Resistance.* Low resistance is important when small infants are allowed to breathe spontaneously. It has to be remembered that the original idea of

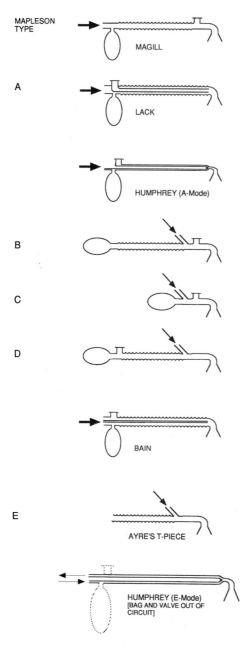

Fig. 3.1 (A–F) Anaesthetic breathing systems for use in children: semi-closed breathing systems. Diagrams show the Mapleson classification of circuits.

B and C are no longer used. Bold arrows indicate fresh gas flow.

Table 3.1

	Full-term neonate	Premature neonate
Weight (kg)	3.5	1.7
Tidal volume (ml)	20	12
Dead space (%)	30	50–60
Alveolar ventilation (ml)	10	6

the system was to avoid rebreathing. Now it is often used with assisted or controlled ventilation with partial rebreathing, carbon dioxide being monitored with a capnograph.

If the open-tail is occluded to keep the bag full, resistance is much increased, and should be borne in mind if a small child is breathing spontaneously.

3. *Humidity.* Dry gases are inhaled through a high flow system and this can damage the activity of cilia in the respiratory tract and reduce mucus formation. It is also associated with significant heat loss which is especially important in neonates and small infants. Artificial humidification is therefore very important and is discussed in a later section.

4. *The bulk of the equipment and tubing.* If the equipment is unwieldy and does not fit together easily there is always a risk of disconnection and kinking. With modern monitoring systems it is essential to have standard fittings (these will be discussed later).

Advantages of the T-piece
- Dead space is very small.
- Minimal resistance (unless the bag is occluded), and no valves.
- Apparatus is simple, compact, and lightweight, and can be disposable.
- Can be used for spontaneous or controlled ventilation.

Disadvantages of the T-piece
- Loss of heat and humidity.
- High flow required (cost implications).
- No pressure relieving safety valve if expiratory tube becomes blocked.
- Difficult to scavenge. Special scavenging attachments are now available (Fig. 3.2c) but increase the resistance to spontaneous respiration.

Spontaneous ventilation with the T-piece
The circuit was originally designed for spontaneous ventilation which requires a fresh gas flow of 2.5 to 3 times the child's minute ventilation.

Controlled ventilation with the T-piece

Since end-tidal CO_2 is now measured using a capnograph it is possible to utilize a partial rebreathing technique. The minimum recommended fresh gas flow required per minute to avoid alveolar rebreathing during controlled ventilation in young children weighing less than 20 kg is 1000 ml + 200 ml kg^{-1}.[3]

The important points to consider are fresh gas flow and minute ventilation. Nightingale et al.[4] concluded that under clinical conditions of mild hyperventilation, a fresh gas flow of 220 ml kg^{-1} is sufficient to prevent hypercapnia. As a result of this work a minimum flow rate of 3 l min^{-1} was recommended for infants and children less than 13.5 kg. However, this does convert the T-piece to a complete non-rebreathing system and with neonates often results in hypocapnia. It is now possible to measure end tidal carbon dioxide (P_ECO_2 in small infants and neonates and the fresh gas flow can be adjusted accordingly, perhaps with the addition of carbon dioxide, although some capnographs do not function well with added carbon dioxide.

The T-piece has now been manufactured in plastic by Portex using both an 8.5 mm and a 15 mm system of connectors. This has considerably reduced the bulk of the equipment and has made the connections much more standardized. 15 mm connectors are the ISO (International Standards Organisation) standard.

The Bain circuit (Mapleson D)

A new coaxial circuit was introduced by Bain and Spoerel in 1972.[5] This is a T-piece system with the fresh gas delivery tube placed inside a lightweight plastic expiratory limb. They recommended that for patients weighing less than 50 kg, the fresh gas flow rate for controlled ventilation should be 70 ml kg^{-1} min^{-1} and this results in an arterial CO_2 (P_aCO_2) of about 40 mm Hg (tidal volume 10 ml kg^{-1}, respiratory rate 10–12 min^{-1}). The same authors[6] concluded that a minimum flow of 3.5 l min^{-1} for children weighing 10–35 kg and a minimum flow of 2 l min^{-1} for infants weighing less than 10 kg were more appropriate. Again with the introduction of capnography more precise control of the fresh gas flow can be made of small infants with, perhaps, the addition of carbon dioxide. Rebreathing does not occur with fresh gas flows of 2–3 times the minute ventilation. Maximum permissible rebreathing occurs with a fresh gas flow in the range of 0.6–1 times the minute volume, but expressed as ml kg^{-1}, minute volume is much higher in infants than in older children and adults.

In very small infants it may be necessary to add carbon dioxide to the fresh gas in order to maintain normocapnia when using a ventilator. This technique relies on accurate flow meters. The CO_2 flow meters on some anaesthetic machines (2 l min^{-1} × 0.1 l min^{-1} graduations) are not appropriate for such small volumes.

gested[9] that with spontaneous ventilation in the 'A' mode and controlled ventilation in the 'D' mode of children weighing less than 20 kg, that fresh gas flows (FGF) need not exceed 3 l min^{-1}. The 'single lever' Humphrey A/E system has been compared with the T-piece during controlled ventilation (E mode) and assessed for efficiency in the 'A' mode by observing the FGF at which rebreathing occurred[10]. This is the only version of the circuit which is now manufactured, a single lever enabling the mode to be changed from A to E.

With the lever in the upright position, the ventilator is out of circuit and the system consists of a reservoir bag, inspiratory limb, and a distal expiratory valve (Fig. 3.3(b)).

This is the 'A' mode. When the lever is moved through 180°, the ventilator is brought into the circuit and the bag is excluded together with the expiratory valve, converting the system to the E configuration.

- Hand ventilation with this circuit is possible only in the 'A' mode. End tidal PCO_2 may rise[10] unless FGF is increased above 3 l min^{-1}.

- Humphrey has shown in adults breathing spontaneously in the 'A' mode that this circuit is actually more efficient than the Magill 'A' system [11] which he attributes to the use of smooth bore tubing and the presence of an 'anvil' in the Y-piece, which tends to split the gas flow and reduce turbulence.

- The expiratory valve has a low opening pressure and dumps increasing amounts of gas with very little increase in resistance, i.e. it is almost linear from 10 to 30 l min^{-1} (airway pressure rises from 1.0 to only 1.3 cm H_2O over the range 10–60 l min^{-1} expiratory flow).

- Thus the valve is not acting as a choke which would cause exponential increase in airway pressure with increasing flow but rather remains closed until 0.8 cm H_2O. Pressure is then applied to the circuit as CPAP or PEEP of around 1.0 to 1.5 cm H_2O which is considered beneficial in small children. This represents an added advantage over spontaneous ventilation with an open T-piece. Scavenging devices (Fig. 3.2c) for the T-piece may significantly increase the work of breathing by increasing resistance to gas flow.

- In order to obtain full advantage from the Humphrey circuit, smooth bore tubing, which minimizes resistance to gas flow, must be used.

- The 15 mm tubing recommended by the manufacturers can be used for both adult and paediatric patients.

- This circuit is certainly suitable for children weighing more than 12 kg. Below this weight the 22 mm Y-piece becomes unwieldy.

CIRCLE SYSTEMS

Low compliance circle systems with lightweight valves are now available and suitable for children weighing more than 20 kg. Conservation of heat and

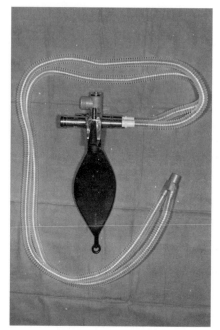

(a)

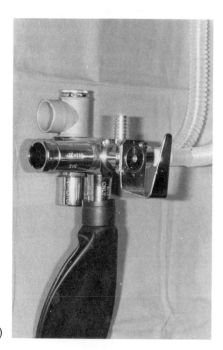

(b)

Fig. 3.3 The Humphrey A/E circuit.

moisture is an advantage, and more economical use of volatile agents may be achieved.

HUMIDIFICATION

Under normal circumstances about 25 per cent of an infant's heat loss is due to evaporation of perspiration or insensible loss from skin and lungs. About one-third of this loss via the lungs. This increases significantly during anaesthesia because inspired anaesthetic gases are dry and at a low ambient temperature. It is therefore important to provide humidified gases in a circuit in order to prevent heat and water loss. This is one of the advantages gained when using a circle system. Heat conservation and humidity are totally lost when using the T-piece system in the non-rebreathing mode.

Humidity can be improved in any anaesthetic breathing system by using either a heat moisture exchanger or a servo controlled heated humidifier.

Heat and moisture exchanger (HME)

These devices humidify inspired gases by capturing and conserving heat and moisture expired from the patient's lungs (see Fig. 3.4). The principle employed is that the latent heat of vaporization/condensation is conserved by the device. A recent refinement of the HME is the hygroscopic condenser humidifier and this contains added hygroscopic material which binds the water molecules in the expired gas. Most of the variants of these devices now employed in anaesthesia also claim to be effective bacterial/viral filters. Hydrophobic membrane filters are the most efficient of these but tend to be bulky and unsuitable for use with small children.

Advantages
- Passive operation: no external source of heat or water required.
- Relatively low cost and disposable.

Disadvantages
- May create unacceptable resistance during inspiration and expiration if the patient is breathing spontaneously.
- May cause an increased inspiratory effort which causes increased heat and water loss.
- Secretions deposited on the humidifier may lead to obstruction.

Their efficiency is quoted as approximately 80 per cent but is often less. The dead space may be significant in a small child but several sizes are available.

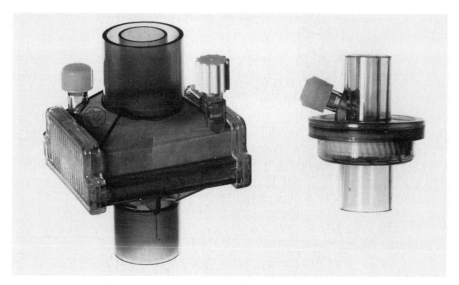

Fig. 3.4 Disposable heat and moisture exchanger filters (HMEFs) with capnograph sampling port.

They should only be used in small children when using intermittent positive pressure ventilation (IPPV).

Servo-controlled humidifier (e.g. Fisher Paykell)

This is a heated water bath humidifier with a heated delivery hose which is servo-controlled (Fig. 3.5). In the past there has always been a problem with any form of water bath due to 'rainout' occurring in the delivery tube to the patient. By using a heated delivery hose this has been eliminated and gases can be delivered to the trachea at 37 °C with up to 99 per cent relative humidity (44 mg l^{-1} water vapour at body temperature). A low compliance chamber is also available for neonates and infants. This humidifier is based on the plenum principle with a large surface area paper wick which is very efficient. It is monitored by thermistors at the hot plate and in the hose.

FACEMASKS AND AIRWAYS

It is important to use a mask with a low deadspace. Such a mask was designed by Rendell-Baker and Soucek[12] and the smallest has a deadspace of 4 ml. They are available in clear plastic as well as rubber and in five sizes (0, 1, 2, 3, 4). For older children, masks with inflatable rims can be used (dead space typically 15 ml). The Rendell-Baker mask is difficult to use

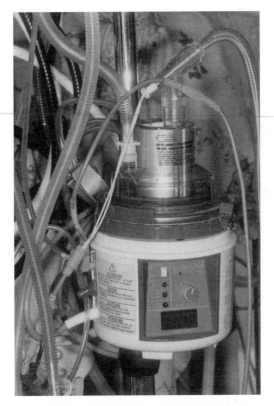

Fig. 3.5 Heated servo-controlled humidifier.

initially but with practice can be used to obtain a complete seal. Oral airways are available in eight sizes (000, 00, 0, 1, 1A, 2, 3, and 4). Use of an oral airway does not always overcome airway obstruction in children, since this is partly due to loss of pharyngeal and laryngeal muscle tone under anaesthesia.

In many neonates and infants they are not usually required and a good airway can be easily managed by careful use of the Rendell-Baker mask, applying the lower edge of the mask between the chin and lower lip with light pressure on the nasal part of the mask. The round Ambu mask is particularly suitable for neonates. (Fig. 3.6b)

ENDOTRACHEAL TUBES

Most endotracheal tubes are now made of polyvinyl chloride (PVC) or polyurethane, and are disposable. They are implantation tested and are marked with the internal and external diameter of the tube. These tubes are routinely used via the nasotracheal route for long-term intubation on the inten-

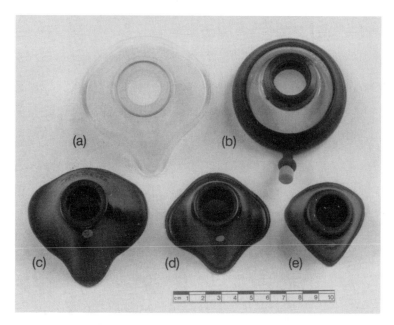

Fig. 3.6 Paediatric face masks. (a,c,d,e) Rendell-Baker and Soucek masks; (b) Ambu mask.

sive care unit and this has encouraged their use for anaesthesia. Any tube inserted into the trachea in children must have a leak around it because of the danger of subglottic damage. The narrowest part of the upper airway in infancy and childhood is the subglottic region, where the complete ring of the cricoid cartilage prevents expansion so that any oedema restricts the airway. Cuffed endotracheal tubes are not often used in children under the age of 10 years.

Tubes can be cut to a specific length for each child. Uncut tubes are more prone to kinking, thereby increasing airway resistance.

Length of oral tube (cm) = internal diameter (mm) × 3 or age/2 + 12 cm.
Internal diameter (mm) = age/4 + 4.0 over 1 year of age.

Some authors do not recommend that tubes should be cut but if they are not, great vigilance is required to ensure that kinking does not occur.

Armoured tubes

Non-kinking tubes (armoured tubes) are also available for children and silicone rubber tubes do not have such a thick wall as reinforced latex tubes which can increase airway resistance. *Preformed* tubes (e.g. RAE) are also available with a nasal or an oral bend.

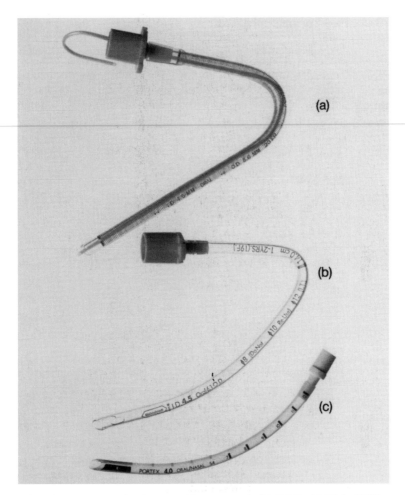

Fig. 3.7 Endotracheal tubes. (a) armoured; (b) RAE; (c) Plain PVC

Connections

The current ISO standard is 15 mm, but is less suitable for small children than the 8.5 mm system as made by Portex.

BRAIN LARYNGEAL MASK AIRWAY: INTAVENT LARYNGEAL MASK (LMA)

There are four sizes available for use in children:

1. neonatal up to 6.5 kg   2–4 ml air in cuff
2. 6.5–25 kg   10 ml air in cuff

Table 3.2   Endotracheal tube sizes

Age	Weight (kg)	Internal diameter (mm)	Length (cm)
Premature	2.5 or less	2.5–3.0	8.5–9.0
Neonate	3	3.0–3.5	9.0–9.5
6 months	6	4.0	10–11.0
1 year	10	4.5	12.0
2 years	12–13	5.0	13.0
3	14–15	5.0	13.5
4	16	5.5	14.0
5	18	5.5	14.5
6	20	6.0	15
7	22	6.0	15.5
8	24	6.5	16.0
9	26–28	6.5	16.5
10	30–32	7.0	17.0
11	32–34	7.0	17.5
12	36	7.5	18.0
13	40	7.5	18.5
14	45+	8.0	19.0
15	50+	8.0	20.0

These sizes are only a guide. Considerable individual variation exists. Tube length is more closely related to age than weight.

Armoured tubes have thicker walls than standard PVC tubes and so one size smaller than indicated in the chart may be required.

$2\frac{1}{2}$. 20–30 kg   up to 14 ml air in cuff

   3. 25 kg to small adult   20 ml air in cuff

These laryngeal masks (Fig. 3.8) should only be used in infants and children once an anaesthetist is totally familiar with the technique in adults. The great danger is that of gastric distension and the mask must not be used for controlled ventilation in small children.

Armoured-tube versions are also available but are sometimes more difficult to insert as the tube is less rigid. These airways cause less circulatory disturbance than an endotracheal tube on insertion and there is less cough and laryngospasm on removal. They have been successfully employed for tonsillectomy and adenoidectomy[13] and to aid fibreoptic intubation in children[14,15]. For a review the reader is referred to Haynes and Morton[16]. A new mask with a double cuff is currently under development which may give a better seal at the oesophagus[17].

LARYNGOSCOPES

Many laryngoscope blades are available for use in small children. The choice of blade is due to the variation in anatomy found in small infants and chil-

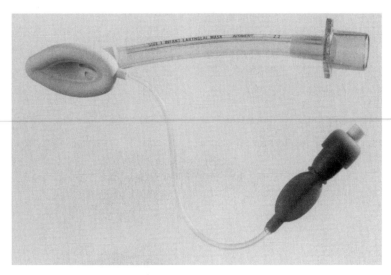

Fig. 3.8 Brain laryngeal mask (Intavent).

dren (Chapter 1). In young children the larynx lies higher and more anteriorly in the neck and the epiglottis is long and thin. The neonatal straight laryngoscope blades are small and do not take up much room in the mouth, and using a straight blade it is possible to lift up the epiglottis to view the larynx. Many different types of straight blades are available, including Robertshaw and Seward (see Fig. 3.9). The use of the different type of straight blade and age at which a change is made to a curved laryngoscope blade is largely an individual choice. For nasal intubation in small children it is important to use a small blade so that the view of the larynx is not obscured when using Magill forceps.

Certain special indirect laryngoscopes may be used in difficult situations to gain an improved view[18].

TYPES OF MECHANICAL VENTILATORS

There are many different types of ventilators available for use in children which can basically be classified into two groups. All the ventilators used are positive pressure ventilators.

Volume or flow control

The main variable is the volume of gas delivered which is satisfactory as long as there are no large leaks in the circuit. In neonates and infants where uncuffed endotracheal tubes are used there is a variable and large leak in the

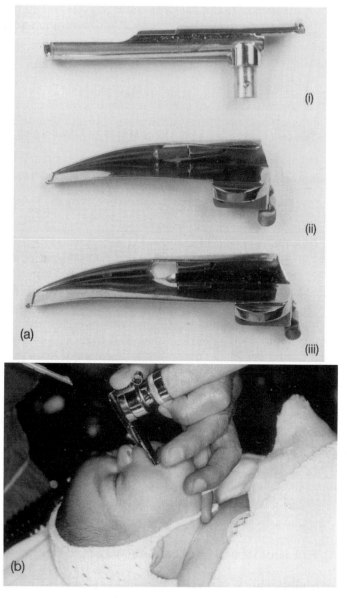

Fig. 3.9 (a) Infant laryngoscopes: (i) Shadwell; (ii) neonatal Robertshaw; (iii) infant Robertshaw. (b) Intubation of small infant. Note neck in neutral position and anaesthetist's little finger applying pressure on the larynx to bring the glottis into view.

circuit. It is also difficult to estimate the volume of gas needed when the tidal volume of the patient is small in comparison to the volume of the ventilator circuitry. It is important to use tubing of low compliance when such ventilators are used for infants with small tidal volumes.

Addition of a plenum humidifier or a circle absorber increases the compliance of the circuit making accurate delivery of small tidal volumes even more difficult.

Pressure control

A pressure controlled ventilator delivers an unspecified volume of gas to the child, but it limits the maximum pressure delivered. The actual alveolar ventilation is unknown and ideally ventilation is monitored by capnography.

Cycling mechanism

In addition to the main variables of pressure or volume, ventilators have different methods of cycling.

1. Pressure cycling delivers gas to the circuit until a preset pressure is reached at which point the inspiratory cycle stops. Using this system it is necessary to be aware of major changes in lung compliance, either due to thoracic or abdominal variations, e.g. a large abdomen pushing the diaphragm up into the chest: decompression at laparotomy will result in airway pressure changes.
2. Time cycling allows the greatest control of the ventilatory cycle. Gas is delivered until a set pressure is reached but the pressure is maintained until a preset inspiratory time is completed, when the cycle finishes.
3. Volume cycling stops inspiration when a preset inspired volume has been delivered.

T-piece occluding ventilators

Ventilation in neonates and small children can be carried out be squeezing the bag on the open limb of an Ayre's T-piece circuit — the 'educated hand'. However, this can easily be replaced by a ventilator that intermittently occludes the end of the limb causing inspiration. Expiration is passively to atmosphere or against a PEEP valve.

A number of ventilators can be used to intermittently occlude the expiratory limb of a T-piece or replace the bag in a Bain circuit.

Originally adult ventilators were modified for use in children but were not always satisfactory. The modification of the Nuffield Anaesthesia ventilator series 200 as described by Newton[19] is ideal for neonatal and paediatric use (Fig. 3.10). It is basically a time cycled constant flow generator converted into a time cycled pressure generator by having a fixed leak (the Newton 'Valve'). It has adjustable inspiratory and expiratory times and can deliver tidal volumes between 10 and 300 ml at frequencies from 10 to 85 min^{-1}. The flow control knob has an adjustment of gas flow from 0.25 to 1.0 l s^{-1} and the pressure developed is shown on a manometer on the front of the

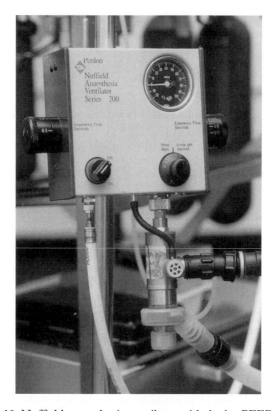

Fig. 3.10 Nuffield anaesthesia ventilator with Ambu PEEP valve.

ventilator. When the Newton valve is in use, much of this gas is not delivered to the patient and those flow markings no longer apply.

Advantages
- It is possible to alter ventilation by changing the inflation pressure.
- Can compensate for leaks around an uncuffed endotracheal tube.
- The fixed leak enables the inspiratory flow rate to be reduced below that of the fresh gas flow (FGF) entering the circuit, thereby delivering the appropriate tidal volume.
- Can use positive end-expiratory pressure.
- Common expiratory outlet is good for scavenging.

Disadvantages
- Noisy — but can be reduced with scavenging.
- A disconnection alarm is essential because the ventilator will continue to function even if disconnected from the patient circuit.

REFERENCES

1. Ayre, P. (1937). Endotracheal anesthesia for babies: with special reference to hare-lip and cleft palate operations. *Anesthesia and Analgesia*, **16**, 330.
2. Harrison, G. A. (1964). Ayre's T-piece; a review of its modifications. *British Journal of Anaesthesia*, **36**, 115.
3. Hatch, D. J., Yates, A. P., and Lindahl, S. G. E. (1987). Flow requirements and rebreathing during mechanically controlled ventilation in T-piece (Mapleson E) systems. *British Journal of Anaesthesia*, **59**, 1533.
4. Nightingale, D. A., Richards, C. C., and Glass, A. (1965). An evaluation of rebreathing in a modified T-piece system during controlled ventilation of anaesthetized children. *British Journal of Anaesthesia*, **37**, 726.
5. Bain, J. A. and Spoerel, W. E. (1972). A streamlined anaesthetic system. *Canadian Anaesthetists' Society Journal*, **19**, 426.
6. Bain, J. A. and Spoerel, W. E. (1977). Carbon dioxide output and elimination in children under anaesthesia. *Canadian Anaesthetists' Society Journal*, **24**, 533.
7. Humphrey, D. and Brocke-Utne, J.G. (1987). Suggested solutions to the problems of the T-piece anaesthetic breathing system. *Canadian Journal of Anaesthesia*, **34**, S129.
8. Humphrey, D. (1983). A new anaesthetic breathing system combining Mapleson A, D and E principles. *Anaesthesia*, **38**, 361.
9. Humphrey, D. and Brock-Utne, J. G. (1985). Lightweight, economical and pollution-free paediatric breathing systems: a new approach. *Acta Anaesthesiologica Scandinavica*, **29**, (Suppl. 80), 65.
10. Orlikowski, C., Ewart, M., and Bingham, R. (1991). The Humphrey ADE system: evaluation in paediatric use. *British Journal of Anaesthesia*, **66**, 253.
11. Humphrey, D., Brock-Utne, J. G. and Downing, J. W. (1986). Single lever Humphrey ADE low flow universal anaesthetic breathing system. Part I: Comparison with dual lever ADE, Magill and Bain Systems in anaesthetised spontaneously breathing adults. *Canadian Anaesthetists Society Journal*, **33**, 710.
12. Rendell-Baker, L. and Soucek, D. M. (1962). New paediatric facemasks and anaesthetic equipment. *British Medical Journal*, **i**, 1690.
13. Dubreuil, M. *et al.* (1993). Is adenoidectomy in children safer with laryngeal mask airway or with tracheal intubation? *Paediatric Anaesthesia*, **3**, 375.
14. White, A. P. and Billingham (1992). Laryngeal mask guided tracheal intubation in paediatric anaesthesia. *Paediatric Anaesthesia*, **2**, 265.
15. Inada, T., Fujise, K., Tachibana, K. *et al.* (1995). Orotracheal intubation through the laryngeal mask airway in patients with Treacher-Collins syndrome. *Paediatric Anaesthesia*, **5**, 129.
16. Maynes, S. K. and Morton, N. S. (1993) The laryngeal mask airway: a review of its use in paediatric anaesthesia. *Paediatric Anaesthesia*, **3**, 65.
17. Brain, A. Y., Verghese, C., Strube, P. *et al.* (1995). A new laryngeal mask prototype. Preliminary investigation of seal pressures and glottic isolation. *Anaesthesia*, **50**, 42.
18. Borland, L.M. and Casselbrant, M. (1990). The Bullard Laryngoscope. A new indirect oral laryngoscope (paediatric version). *Anesthesia and Analgesia*, **70**, 105.
19. Newton, N. I., Hillman, K. M., and Varley, S. G. (1981). Automatic ventilation with the Ayre's T-piece. A modification of the Nuffield series 200 ventilator for neonatal and paediatric use. *Anaesthesia*, **36**, 22.

4

Monitoring in paediatric anaesthesia

D. G. Hughes

Observation of a patient's skin colour, that of the mucous membranes, and regular palpation of the peripheral pulse are simple yet useful methods of monitoring the patient during anaesthesia.

SIMPLE CLINICAL OBSERVATION

It is important in paediatric anaesthesia to monitor a child by continuous clinical observations. This involves most of the five senses but visual observation of the patient will provide the most useful information. It is very easy to observe the colour of the skin and blood; any abnormal respiratory pattern should be detected long before changes occur on the sophisticated monitors on which anaesthetists now rely. A well-completed anaesthetic chart will enable down or upward trends in any of the vital parameters to be immediately observed and will also act as a medicolegal document. The extra observations that need to be recorded in paediatric practice include temperature and fluid balance and it is also useful to record the effect that the premedication or pre-operative visit has had on the child.

CARDIOVASCULAR MONITORING

Stethoscope

The heart rate and rhythm can be continuously monitored by auscultation using a precordial or oesophageal stethoscope (Fig. 4.1). This can be attached by a long tube (at least 120 cm) to normal stethoscope earpieces or can be connected to a monaural ear piece which can be kept in the anaesthetist's ear during an operation. The precordial stethoscope must be firmly fixed to the chest wall with an adhesive disc or tape. The smallest available oesophageal stethoscope is 8FG. The stethoscope is inserted into the oesophagus until maximum heart sounds are heard. It is then possible to monitor the heart rate continuously and listen to the breath sounds, although observation of chest wall movement is essential to ensure that ventilation is proceeding at preset levels.

Table 4.1   Monitoring in young children

Simple clinical observations:
Colour of skin and mucous membranes,
peripheral pulses, chest excursion,
respiratory rate and rhythm

Cardiovascular monitoring
Stethoscope (oesophageal or precordial)
Electrocardiogram
Blood pressure
   Non-invasive
   Invasive
Central venous pressure

Respiratory monitoring
Breathing — pattern or ventilator parameters
Blood gases
   Non-invasive
   Invasive

Fluid balance
Fluid input
Urine output
Insensible loss (estimate)
Blood loss/secretions (e.g. nasogastric aspirate)

Temperature

Neuromuscular function

Electrocardiogram

The electrocardiogram (ECG) provides the anaesthetist with information about the heart rate and its rhythm, the site of abnormal pacemakers, and the efficiency of the conducting tissues. Its most important function in infants and children is the detection of bradycardia, since children rarely develop other dysrhythmias and do not frequently suffer from diseases of the myocardium. However, in children with much faster heart rates (180 beats min^{-1}) and smaller chest diameters, a number of problems may arise. The ECG can be monitored using the same lead systems as adults and preferably should be interchangeable with an Intensive Care Unit or a Special Care Baby Unit system. The electrodes must be smaller, more flexible, and very adhesive.

With the rapid heart rates found in children, and since the electrodes are close together, the T wave may become nearly as large as the QRS complex, resulting in false readings of the heart rate. This can be offset by using an adjustable gain. It may also be necessary to increase the sweep rate from 25 mm sec^{-1} to 50 mm sec^{-1} to assist in the analysis of the waveform. The response of neonates and small infants to hypoxaemia is bradycardia. Children are also prone to develop bradycardia following the use of suxamethonium and halothane.

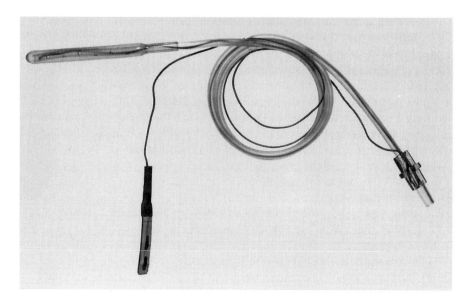

Fig. 4.1 Oesophageal stethoscope with thermistor.

It must be remembered that a relatively normal tracing can still be obtained when the heart has ceased to beat effectively as a pump (electromechanical dissociation; EMD) and an ECG should always be used in conjunction with a monitor of the peripheral circulation such as an oximeter, a pulse monitor, or an oscillotonometer.

Blood pressure monitoring

Blood pressure should always be monitored in children because the peripheral vascular resistance and myocardial contractility of children are markedly affected by anaesthetic agents. Normal heart rates and blood pressures for infants and children are given in Chapter 2. Blood pressure can be measured using either non-invasive or invasive techniques.

Non-invasive monitoring

There are many non-invasive techniques available for the measurement of arterial blood pressure and these include flush, palpatory, auscultatory, oscillotonometric, and Doppler methods. Flush and palpatory methods are critically dependent upon the technique and skill of the operator and are not sufficiently accurate to justify continued use. Auscultatory methods depend upon the presence of Korotkoff sounds which are frequently unobtainable in infants. For many years the Doppler method of blood pressure determination has been found to be consistently accurate even under hypotensive conditions. These devices detect sound waves that are reflected from moving arterial walls. The ultrasonic measurement of blood pressure depends on the use of an occlusion cuff and an ultrasonic transducer usually placed over the brachial artery. The transducer consists of an ultrasonic signal generator and a receiver. The change in frequency associated with vessel wall movement is used to record systolic and diastolic blood pressures. The output from the transducer is amplified and filtered and may be used to produce an audible signal or a printed record. However, for the clinical anaesthetist working in a noisy operating theatre it has many disadvantages, including the need for accurate placement over the artery, and an ultrasonic coupling gel. It is also susceptible to motion and accidental displacement by surgical colleagues.

In the late 1970s improved automated blood pressure devices based on the oscillometric principle (Dinamap) became available for the measurement of systolic, mean, diastolic pressures, and heart rates in adults. New technology enabled this system to be used in neonates and children in the early 1980s. Probably the most important determinant of blood pressure in smaller infants is the size of the cuff in relation to arm circumference. The importance of this was demonstrated by Kimble *et al.*[1] They looked at different cuff sizes and took 10 determinations for each cuff on each infant. Their readings were compared with direct readings of intra-arterial values of blood pressure. They suggested that minimal error was found when the ratio of cuff width to arm circumference was within the range of 0.45–0.7. Similar results were shown by Pelligrini-Calium *et al.*[2]

A number of studies have been carried out to evaluate the use of these oscillometric devices in neonates and infants but have been mainly carried out on sedated infants in a special care baby unit or in the cardiac catheter laboratory. These relatively stable environments bear little resemblance to the marked fluctuations in blood pressure commonly seen during clinical anaesthesia and surgery. Friesen and Lichtor[3] in their study comparing oscillometric readings with intra-arterial readings, took five readings in 20 neonates/infants during anaesthesia, prior to surgery, and found the Dinamap to be an accurate monitor for this age group. Cullen *et al.* carried out a similar study with a larger group of patients (again comparing with direct arterial pressure) and found the Dinamap to be an excellent indicator of heart rate.[4] As an indicator of systolic pressure it under-reads at high arterial pressures and over-reads at low pressures. The mean arterial pressure was consistently higher than the intra-arterial values. The Dinamap has been found to be an accurate trend recorder of blood pressure and heart rate during anaesthesia in small infants.

Ideally, in order to minimize the overall error, several consecutive measurements should be performed and their average value taken. Care must be taken to ensure that cycling is not too frequent in neonates and small infants because of the risk of damage to the limb.

Invasive monitoring

Invasive monitoring of the arterial blood pressure is often required in the operating theatre when large fluid or blood losses are anticipated or hypotensive anaesthesia is being employed. This use of arterial catheterization enables frequent arterial blood sampling to be successfully carried out with minimal disturbance to the child. Percutaneous catheterization is possible in most arteries and the site chosen is usually determined by the operative technique and the possible complications that may arise. The sites used have included the radial, ulnar, brachial, femoral, dorsalis pedis, and posterior tibial arteries. For long-term use clinicians prefer to avoid using the femoral artery for monitoring except in cardiac patients. The radial artery is the most favoured site for cannulation and the technique described for the approach can be used for all other arteries. In premature infants and neonates, Cole *et al.* have described a method of locating arteries using a bright cold fibreoptic light.[5] This technique is now widely used. The cannula in small infants is inserted percutaneously using a technique whereby the artery is transfixed, slow withdrawal until blood is visualized, and then the catheter is advanced over the needle into the artery. A 22 or 24 gauge Teflon catheter is preferred. In older children it is not necessary to transfix the artery and the catheter can be advanced as soon as blood flows into the hub of the needle. A catheter with wings is used because it can be very easily fixed to an arm or leg. Adequate skin puncture should be made prior to cannulation otherwise the catheter will peel back. Occasionally it may be necessary to use a Seldinger technique, similar to that used for percutaneous central venous lines. In certain operations it is important to cannulate the right brachial or radial artery, and these include coarctation of the aorta, left Blalock–Taussig shunt, patent ductus arteriosus, and diaphragmatic herniae (i.e. in the pre-ductal site).

The catheter is connected to a three-way tap with Luer locks. There will be an increased risk of infection with the stopcock and special care needs to be observed when blood samples are taken. The line is connected to a pressure transducer through non-compliant tubing and is maintained patent by using a continuous flush with 0.45% saline + 1 unit heparin ml^{-1}. By using an infusion pump through a continuous flush device it is possible to adjust the flow between 0.5 and 3 ml h^{-1}. The flush device also isolates the transducer from the pump and so reduces artefacts and any damping effects produced by the syringe pump.

In the operating theatre it is important to position the sampling tap so that it is readily accessible. The manometer tubing should be short because of its effects on the frequency response, since many infants have a rapid heart rate (3 Hz). Both the connectors and the puncture site should be visible at all times and should be covered with an occlusive plastic dressing. The lines should be clearly labelled ARTERIAL.

The other arteries used, including the brachial, dorsalis pedis, and posterior tibial artery, are frequently cannulated without any special problems being reported. The femoral artery is often used in cardiac surgery although cases of gangrene have been reported when the femoral artery was used for long-term monitoring.[6] However, many of these cases date back to the mid

1960s and one could well speculate that with modern techniques and materials this particular route may not be as hazardous as was previously thought. Perhaps in view of the close proximity to the hip joint and to urine and faeces, it is best not to cannulate this artery for long-term monitoring. Cardiologists now routinely catheterize the femoral artery with 5F gauge catheters for short-term investigations with a low incidence of complications.

Arterial sampling should be carried out with extreme care and slowly to avoid damage to the intima of the artery and any volume of blood taken should be recorded. Flushing of an arterial line should be done with small volumes using a 5 ml syringe. Lowenstein *et al.* have demonstrated that it is possible to inject clots and damaged cells not only into the extremities but also retrogradely into central cerebral vessels.[7] The authors visualized the carotid arteries of children with 1 ml of dye rapidly injected into the radial arteries. A similar picture can be seen when dye is rapidly injected into umbilical artery catheters.

The complication rate for arterial monitoring in children has been well documented. There are many minor sequelae but few major problems.[8] The rare major complications can be avoided by careful observation of the limb. Minor complications at the site of the catheter include haemorrhage, haematoma, and infection. Miyasaska found that obstruction to the radial artery was common in children after removal of the catheter (71 per cent) but permanent obstruction was rare.[9] It is also difficult to carry out an Allen's test in small infants. The embolization described by Lowenstein is a problem and it is not uncommon to see skin blanching on the forearm when a radial catheter is over-zealously flushed. If this persists or if too large a volume of flush is used, permanent damage to skin and muscle can occur. In view of these findings it is probably unwise to use the temporal artery for cannulation. If there is any serious deterioration in colour or marked temperature change in the hand, the catheter must be removed immediately. Rarely is it necessary to carry out surgical exploration for possible embolization.

In neonates it is easy to cannulate the umbilical artery in the first 48 h of life, but there is considerable morbidity associated with this technique including renal, visceral, and lower limb sequelae.

The monitoring equipment used in children must be capable of responding to fast heart rates, sometimes up to 3–4 Hz. Most monitors incorporate several scales to accommodate the different pressure levels. The waveform should be critically examined following a small but rapid flush of the cannula to exclude the presence of 'ringing' due to an over-resonant system.

Central venous pressure (CVP)

The demand for good access to central veins in children has increased steadily and with improved techniques available many routes previously thought to be dangerous in small infants are being routinely used. In many cases central catheters are inserted due to the lack of peripheral venous access and the monitoring of central venous pressure becomes an adjunct in the management of the critically ill child, both during surgery in the operating theatre and in the Intensive Care Unit. Such a cannula provides information on the filling volume of the venous system and the function of the myocardium and can be used for intravenous nutrition and drug administration. Unless children have an associated cardiac defect there is usually a good correlation between right and left ventricular performance. The pressure in the right atrium (RAP) reflects the right ventricular preload or venous capacitance and is not a measure of blood volume. If the central venous pressure is low with a low cardiac output it is appropriate to administer intravenous fluid to give sufficient circulating volume. However, a high central venous pressure is open to more errors in interpretation, especially if the child is on a ventilator. With a high intrathoracic pressure it may be necessary to temporarily disconnect the patient from the ventilator to determine the CVP and the size of the liver. A true high central venous pressure may represent volume overload or loss of right ventricular function. Children with congenital heart disease such as pulmonary stenosis or ventricular septal defects may have isolated right ventricular failure with a high central venous pressure. A similar condition can occur after cardiac surgery involving the right ventricular outflow tract, e.g. pulmonary stenosis and tetralogy of Fallot. It is also possible to have high CVP readings secondary to increases in pulmonary vascular resistance commonly seen in some premature infants.

Catheters are usually inserted percutaneously and should be positioned in a large vein with the tip at the junction of the superior vena cava and the right atrium. Access to this site can be gained by a number of different routes but preferably via the internal jugular or subclavian veins.

Routes of central venous access

- Peripheral arm vein — this is not a reliable route in small children.
- Femoral vein
- Internal jugular vein — the landmarks are less well defined for this route in children. It is reliable and has low morbidity. However, the success rate with this technique is lower than in adults and fixation can be a problem.[10]

    Technique. The child is placed in the head down position with the head turned away from the site of the catheter insertion and a small support placed under the shoulders. The approach is similar to that used for adults. In smaller children the line of direction is usually midway between the ipsilateral nipple and the sternum and the procedure is best carried out using a Seldinger technique.

- Subclavian vein — the infraclavicular approach to this vein has been used in infants and children with varying results. However, for long-term feeding, drug administration, and monitoring it is easier to fix, more comfortable for the child, and not subject to continuous movement. The technique was condemned by many authors.[11] However, the use of a Seldinger technique has enabled this approach to be successfully carried out even in very small neonates.[12] The final position of the catheter is not as reliable as the internal jugular approach, catheters frequently travelling cephalad in the neck vessels.

Technique. Adopting a similar patient position to that used for an internal jugular catheter the point of entry is immediately below the midpoint of the clavicle. The approach is similar to that used in adults except in infants and neonates. In this group the direction of the cannula is more cephalad, about 1–1.5 cm above the suprasternal notch. The final position of the catheter tip must be immediately confirmed by chest radiography. Double lumen catheters are now available for use in children but the smallest size is 18 g (lumen 30/17).

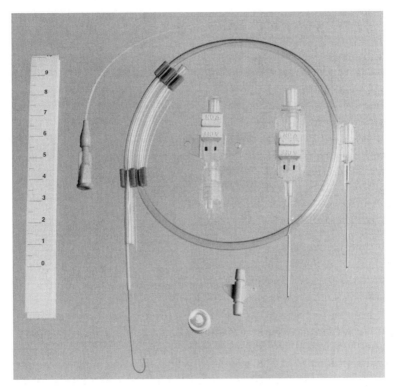

Fig. 4.2 Apparatus for central venous cannulation using Seldinger technique.

RESPIRATORY MONITORING

Breathing

Commercially produced 'apnoea' alarms are available which detect chest wall movement by sensing pressure changes in a small capsule which is applied to the child's body wall using adhesive tape. Each breath may be signalled by a flashing light or an audible 'bleep'. Apnoea beyond a preset delay time will sound an alarm. Their main drawback is that they detect attempted breathing rather than actual air movement to and from the lungs.

A reliable breathing monitor should produce a signal based upon air movement. This may be done by recording changes in carbon dioxide or temperature at the nose, mouth, or endotracheal tube. Air movement in the trachea or lungs can be monitored by a stethoscope placed in the oesophagus or on the precordium.

Blood gases

Arterial blood gas tensions may be monitored either invasively or non-invasively.

Both oxygen and carbon dioxide tensions can be monitored during surgery and in the intensive care unit. Detection of excessively high or low values is especially important in the neonate where high arterial oxygen levels are a factor in retinopathy of prematurity, and low arterial carbon dioxide levels may produce problems with the control of breathing postoperatively.

Invasive blood gas and pH measurement (arterial blood gas, ABG).

Samples may be taken from an indwelling arterial cannula if it is available or an artery may be 'stabbed' with a 25 or 27 gauge needle attached to a heparinized syringe. Most blood gas analysers now require only a small sample of blood and it is important not to over-heparinize the sample as the pH of heparin solution will alter the measured blood pH.

Shunts may occur which affect the arterial oxygen tension (PaO_2) as measured from different sampling sites. For example, in the case of 'transitional' or 'persistent fetal' circulation (see p. 8), there is a right to left shunt through a patient ductus arteriosus. This is usually due to a combination of high pulmonary vascular resistance and hypoxaemia. The effect is for pulmonary arterial blood (unsaturated) to mix with better oxygenated blood in the descending aorta, thus reducing the PaO_2 in the lower body arteries as compared with the right subclavian artery and its branches. By comparing the upper and lower body PaO_2 over a period of time, any increase or decrease in the shunt may be followed. In conditions such as congenital diaphragmatic hernia this can be an invaluable guide to therapy.

Interpretation of blood gases in infants and children follows the same principles as in adults. It is noteworthy that very low pH values of 6.8–7.0 are much more likely to be associated with a complete recovery in neonates than in older patients. Arterial carbon dioxide tensions in neonates are approximately the same as in children and adults but neonates have a low arterial oxygen tension (50–60 mmHg). These values are normal and are associated with high saturation figures because of the high proportion of fetal haemoglobin (HbF). At term the proportion of HbF to HbA in neonatal blood is approximately 80:20. The low P_{50} (see p. 7) of this blood of approximately 19 mm Hg is due in part to a lack of sensitivity of HbF to the effect of 2,3-diphosphoglycerate (2,3-DPG).

Because of the difficulties in obtaining good arterial blood samples from some infants, 'arterialized' capillary blood samples (obtained from a warmed limb), may be used. The CO_2 tension will however be slightly higher than from an arterial sample and the oxygen tension may be considerably lower.

Non-invasive blood gas measurement; Transcutaneous blood gas measurement

Except in cyanotic heart disease, a well-oxygenated paediatric patient should look pink, and constant vigilance on the part of the anaesthetist cannot be exchanged for total reliance on 'high tech' monitors.

Neonates and infants have thin skins with a very good capillary blood supply. Electrodes are available which will continuously measure both transcutaneous oxygen tension ($TcPO_2$) and transcutaneous carbon dioxide tension ($TcPCO_2$) Clinical experience is greater with $TcPO_2$ although combined units are now available.[13]

Transcutaneous electrodes rely upon producing heat-induced vasodilatation in order to achieve maximal accuracy. The required temperature of 43–44 °C is high enough to produce thermal damage to the skin, so great care is needed in their use. Oxygen and carbon dioxide diffuse through the skin to the electrode and appropriate electrical signals are produced which are proportional to their partial pressures. These signals are then processed and displayed by the associated monitors.

$TcPO_2$ monitors are subject to a number of errors. $TcPO_2$ commonly underestimates PaO_2 and this disparity increases with the age of the patient. Trends in oxygenation are, however, well interpreted. Hypotension and poor skin perfusion may produce underestimation of PaO_2. Direct pressure on the electrode also causes under-reading. If the adhesive film attaching the electrode to the patient's skin becomes partially detached, environmental air may gain access to the electrode which will no longer accurately reflect the patient's PO_2. Halothane and nitrous oxide may be chemically reduced and produce a falsely high $TcPO_2$ reading. This effect is minimized by electrodes using a relatively low polarization voltage (<600 mV). The effects of other volatile agents on accuracy are probably less important.

The necessity to change the position of the electrode on the infant's skin every 2–3 h is more of an inconvenience than a major disadvantage. As the skin begins to blister, heat transfer from the electrode to the capillary circulation is reduced, thus less heating is required to maintain electrode temperature. Some monitors incorporate a heating power meter and will signal this as a warning that the site must be changed.

TcPCO_2 systems are subject to fewer inaccuracies and anaesthetic agents have no effect, perfusion and blood pressure are less important, but air can still get underneath a poorly attached electrode.

Systems have been devised for extracting gas from the surface of the skin and analysing it with a mass spectrometer (MS). The problems of sampling are similar to those with the above systems, but because of the specificity of MS analysis there should be no confusion caused by anaesthetic agents, indeed these can be monitored using the MS.

Pulse oximetry

The last few years have seen a surge of interest in this non-invasive technique as a number of manufacturers have produced reliable units.[14] These provide a continuous read-out of arterial oxygen saturation (SaO_2) and of pulse rate. Many pulse oximeters provide a beat-to-beat indication of peripheral pulse by audible or visible means.

Microprocessor technology enables the pulse oximeter to consider only the pulsatile (arterial) elements of light absorption thus ignoring the effects of the tissues and non-pulsatile (venous) blood. The pulse oximeter integrates the physiological principles of plethysmography and oximetry by means of solid-state electronics to provide a continuous monitor of arterial oxygenation. The sensor consists of two light-emitting diodes and a phototransistor detector. It utilizes two wavelengths of light at 660 and 940 nm and an integrated microprocessor-based computer program to measure arteriolar pulsation. Through expansion and relaxation, the pulsating vascular bed changes the length of the light path, thereby modifying the amount of light detected.

Different sensors are available for different monitoring sites (Fig. 4.3). In younger children, the finger and ear may be convenient, but because of their small size it is very common to monitor babies with a flexible probe on either a hand or foot.

Although the pulse oximeter provides a large amount of very useful non-invasive data, it will not detect hyperoxia evidenced by a very high PaO_2 and should ideally be used as a means of detecting hypoxia rather than for indirectly reflecting arterial oxygen tension.[15]

End tidal gas analysis

With suitable equipment, carbon dioxide, oxygen, nitrous oxide, and volatile anaesthetic agents may be monitored on a breath-by-breath basis.

The measurement of the end tidal carbon dioxide concentration or partial pressure (P_ECO_2) in the expired air of fit young adults can be taken to be a good reflection of the arterial carbon dioxide tension P_aCO_2. Because of the

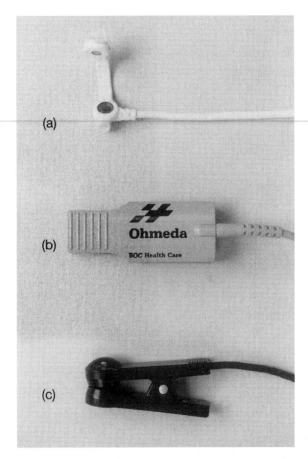

Fig. 4.3 Oximeter probes: (a) neonatal; (b) finger probe; (c) ear clip.

size of the capnograph sampling cells and the high flow rates necessary to obtain a good time response, the application of adult capnographic techniques to paediatric anaesthesia has met with many difficulties. However, there are capnographs available which have either a small analysing cell requiring a reduced gas sampling rate or which are placed in-line in the expiratory limb of the breathing system and possess a low dead space (Hewlett Packard). It is important to ensure that an end tidal plateau is being reached with each breath. A chart recorder or a capnograph which displays a waveform should be used.

The site of sampling from the breathing system is important. It has been shown that sampling from the proximal end of the endotracheal tube is satisfactory.[16] Some capnographs also incorporate an oxygen analyser. If this is of the fuel cell type it will record only an 'average' oxygen concentration. If a paramagnetic oxygen analyser is incorporated, inspired and expired concentrations may be monitored on a breath-to-breath basis and can be used to warn against impending hypoxia.

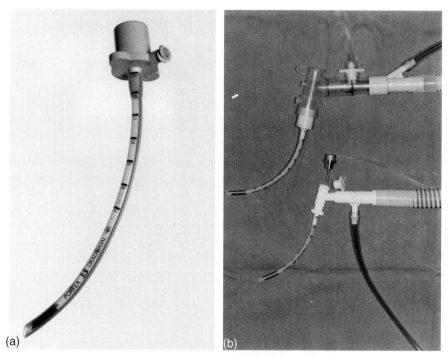

(a)   (b)

Fig. 4.4 (a) 15 mm endotracheal tube connector with sampling port; (b) sampling system for the 8.5 mm mini-link system consisting of a stainless steel plug bearing a 1 mm tube sampling from the tracheal tube connector compared with a standard 15 mm connector and sidestream capnograph attachment.

Lindahl *et al.* have also demonstrated the close relationship between arterial ($PaCO_2$) and end-tidal carbon dioxide (P_ECO_2) in normal infants and children.[17]

Clinical applications include:

- establishing mechanical ventilation;
- monitoring mechanical ventilation — disconnection, leaks, obstruction, ventilator malfunction;
- as an aid to monitoring the circulation (particularly for air embolism);
- weaning from mechanical ventilation.

FLUID BALANCE

A record must be kept of the amount of intravenous fluid given to a small child or infant. Fluid is always given using a calibrated device such as a burette or, as in many centres, the appropriate volume of fluid is delivered either through a syringe pump for very small neonates or through a volumetric infusion pump. In long operations it may be necessary to measure urine output hourly and this can be carried out using a urine collection bag, or in difficult cases with an indwelling catheter connected to a sterile closed draining system. This then becomes an aid to assessing renal function.

BLOOD LOSS

Blood loss has always been difficult to measure in small children and many different ways have been used in an attempt to accurately measure the loss. Weighing of swabs is routine and this can give a reasonably accurate assessment. Although the commonly employed method is to equate 1 g with 1 ml of blood, the true value will vary with the haematocrit. Any blood lost through suction can be measured in a calibrated suction jar. The volumes of blood lost should be recorded at frequent intervals on a wall chart. An accurate record of input and output should be made on the anaesthetic chart since it is very easy to over-transfuse a small infant.

TEMPERATURE MONITORING

The dangers of inadvertent hypothermia in neonates and malignant hyperpyrexia in all children make temperature monitoring essential in paediatric practice. Heat is lost from the body surface by radiation, convection, conduction, and evaporation, including important evaporative and convective heat losses from the airways. The reduction of heat loss is based on two important principles:

- reducing external temperature gradients using heated blankets, increasing the air temperature of the operating theatre, and warming inspired gases;
- reducing the amount of body surface available for heat loss using head coverings and warm gamgee blankets or bubble wrap. The heat lost from the airway can be reduced by using heat and moisture exchangers and can be eliminated totally by using heated humidifiers to warm the inspired gases. These may even add heat and should be kept at 32–37 °C to avoid respiratory tract burns. Preoperative care of the child's temperature, especially in infants, and immediately postoperatively are as important as the intraoperative temperature maintenance, more so if an infant has to be transferred in an incubator.

The modern thermistor probe is very easy to use and the temperature of the child can be monitored in a number of different sits. The nasopharyngeal and oesophageal sites are commonly used but can be affected by the temper-

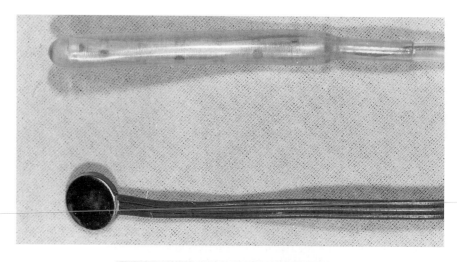

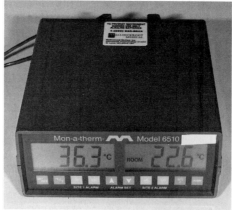

Fig. 4.5 (*above*) Oesophageal stethoscope with temperature probe and skin temperature probe; (*below*) temperature displays

ature of the inspired gases. The axilla, if the probe is properly positioned, can be useful in some operations. Bladder temperature can be monitored using a special urinary catheter which includes a temperature probe and is a good guide to core temperature. The rectal route is rarely used because of the complications associated with this, including slow equilibration of temperature changes and perforation of the rectum. Tympanic membrane probes are improving all the time and this is often thought of as the most accurate measurement of core temperature.

Benzinger has shown that temperature measurement made using the rectal, oesophageal, and axillary sites differs only slightly from tympanic membrane temperature.[18] Trends in temperature monitoring are more important than single observations in order that appropriate measures can be taken to either provide more heat or even turn down heating devices.

Peripheral skin temperature monitoring is only routinely used in cardiac cases and in the intensive care unit where core/peripheral temperature gradients give useful information about peripheral perfusion.

Any piece of apparatus that is used to warm a patient must have its temperature monitored, including water blankets, air heated blankets, and the inspired anaesthetic gases if they are humidified using a heated device.

NEUROMUSCULAR MONITORING

Since the introduction of shorter acting non-depolarizing muscle relaxants, clinicians have used these drugs for continuous infusion during long operative procedures and in intensive care. As a result, more importance has been placed on the ability to accurately monitor neuromuscular function during anaesthesia and to measure signs of recovery.

The basis of the technique is to electrically stimulate a peripheral nerve and visually observe or graphically measure the response of the skeletal muscle supplied by that nerve using evoked mechanical or electromyographic (EMG) response. Usually a surface electrode is placed over the ulnar nerve and the train-of-four (TOF) response of the adductor pollicis brevis is observed by

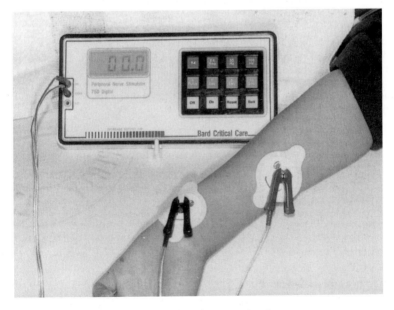

Fig. 4.6 Peripheral nerve stimulator.

applying a supramaximal stimulus using a peripheral nerve stimulator.[19-21] In our department, the Bard Critical Care nerve stimulator has been found satisfactory for clinical use. Newer techniques, such as double burst stimulation, are now entering paediatric anaesthetic practice.

REFERENCES

1. Kimble, K. J. *et al.* (1981). An automated oscillometric technique for estimating mean arterial pressure in critically ill newborn. *Anesthesiology*, **54**, 423.
2. Pelligrini-Calium, G. *et al.* (1982). Evaluation of an automated oscillometric method and various cuffs for the measurement of arterial pressure in the neonate. *Acta Paediatrica Scandinavica*, **71**, 791.
3. Friesen, R. H. and Lichtor, J. L. (1981). Indirect measurement of blood pressure in neonates and infants utilizing an automated non-invasive oscillometric monitor. *Anesthesia and Analgesia*, **60**, 741.
4. Cullen, P. M., Dye, J., and Hughes, D. G. (1987). Clinical assessment of the neonatal Dinamap 847 during anaesthesia in neonates and infants. *Journal of Clinical Monitoring*, **3**, 229.
5. Coe, F. S., Todres, I. D., and Shannon, D. C. (1978). Techniques for percutaneously cannulation of the radial artery in the newborn infant. *Journal of Pediatrics*, **99**, 105.
6. Adams, J. M. and Randolph, A. J. (1975). The use of indwelling radial artery catheters in neonates. *Pediatrics*, **55**, 261.
7. Lowenstein, E., Little, J. W., and Lo, H. H. (1971). Prevention of cerebral embolization from flushing radial artery cannulae. *New England Journal of Medicine*, **285**, 1414.
8. Smith-Wright, D. L. *et al.* (1984). Complications of vascular catheterization in critically ill children. *Critical Care Medicine*, **12**, 1015.
9. Miyasaska, K., Edmonds, J. F., and Conn, A. W. (1979). Complication of radial artery line in the paediatric patient. *Canadian Anaesthetists' Society Journal*, **23**, 9.
10. Nicholson, S. C. *et al.* (1985). Comparison of internal and external jugular cannulation of the central circulation in the paediatric patient. *Critical Care Medicine*, **13**, 747.
11. Prince, S. R., Sullivan, P. L., and Hactiel, A. (1976). Percutaneous cannulation of the internal jugular vein in infants and children. *Anesthesiology*, **44**, 170.
12. Huttel, M. S., Chistensen, P., and Olesen, A. J. (1985). Subclavian venous catheterization in children. *Acta Anaesthesiologia Scandinavica*, **29**, 733.
13. Tremper, K. K. (1984). Transcutaneous PO_2 measurement. *Canadian Anaesthetists' Society Journal*, **31**, 664.
14. Taylor, M. B. and Whitwam, J. G. (1986). The current status of pulse oximetry. *Anesthesia* **41**, 943.
15. Wimberley, P. D. *et al.* (1987). Pulse oximetry versus transcutaneous PO_2 in sick newborn infants. *Scandinavian Journal of Clinical and Laboratory Investigations*, **47**, 19.
16. Stokes, M. A., Hughes, D. G., and Hutton P. (1986). Capnography in the small subject. *British Journal of Anaesthesia*, **58**, 814.

17. Lindahl, S. G. E., Yates, A. P., and Hatch, D. J. (1987). Relationship between invasive and non-invasive measurements of gas exchange in anaesthetized infants and children. *Anesthesiology*, **66**, 168.

18. Benzinger, M. (1969). Tympanic thermometry in surgery and anesthesia. *Journal of the American Medical Association*, **209**, 1207.

19. Viby-Mogensen, J. (1982). Clinical assessment of neuromuscular transmission. *British Journal of Anaesthesia*, **54**, 209.

20. Pither, C. E., Prithvi-Raj, Q., and Ford, D. J. (1985). The use of peripheral nerve stimulators for regional anaesthesia. *Regional Anesthesia*, **10**, 239.

21. Carter, J. A. *et al.* (1986). Assessment of the Datex Relaxograph during anaesthesia and atracurium-induced neuromuscular blockade. *British Journal of Anaesthesia*, **58**, 1447.

5

Basic concepts of paediatric anaesthesia practice

S. J. Mather

PRE-OPERATIVE ASSESSMENT

Before deciding what sort of anaesthetic technique to use, the anaesthetist must consider the following:

- the proposed operation and whether it is elective or an emergency;
- its timing in relation to the last meal or drink;
- the physical status of the patient, including any congenital malformations;
- if the patient is less than 6 months of age, whether prematurity is a factor;
- what the child's weight is;
- in the neonatal period the birth weight, gestation, and progress since birth (e.g. has ventilation been required for respiratory distress syndrome);
- family history (e.g. sickle-cell disease);
- previous surgery or anaesthesia;
- recent respiratory tract infection;
- the results of laboratory investigations;
- current medication.

THE PROPOSED OPERATION

The site which is to be operated upon may dictate which type of technique is to be preferred, for example head and neck surgery will almost always require intubation, especially in babies, or the use of a laryngeal mask airway. Certain operations require muscle relaxation which will necessitate intubation for positive pressure ventilation.

Elective procedures enable one to plan an anaesthetic at leisure, and to consult reference textbooks if necessary for information about rarer diseases. Emergency surgery leaves one little time for preparation or assessment. Only exceptionally, however, is it necessary to operate before the results of haematological or biochemical investigations are available and adequate resuscitation has been carried out.

THE LAST MEAL OR DRINK

This often causes controversy, but may dictate the time at which elective surgery can proceed. In the older child who has not been traumatized or treated with opioids, one can expect the stomach to be empty within 4 h. Anxiety delays gastric emptying. Neonates and small infants empty more quickly and 3 h starvation is regarded by many as safe.[1]

In reality, however, the stomach is never truly empty and can not be completely emptied even via a gastric tube. If blood is present, clots should be washed out if possible through a large bore tube and the tube left on free drainage. In trauma patients, one must expect that the stomach will contain undigested food.[2] Pharmacologically induced vomiting should never be contemplated since aspiration may occur. A rapid-sequence induction using cricoid pressure is safe and effective.

Authors vary in their recommendations for pre-operative starvation. Long periods of starvation, in excess of 6 h, may lead to glycogen depletion and ketosis in stressed babies. If prolonged starvation is contemplated for any reason, intravenous 5 or 10 per cent glucose should be given to small children. (Administration of glucose during the operation may, however, cause *hyperglycaemia* and frequent monitoring of blood glucose is required.) Rarely, hypoglycaemia may occur in older children after routine pre-operative fasting.[3]

On balance, a starvation period of 4 h for older children and 3 h for milk (possibly 2 h for clear fluids) in neonates and infants seems reasonable. Expediency for the sake of convenience on operating lists must be resisted.

Metoclopramide has been advocated to increase the rate of gastric emptying but it is ineffective in many cases (especially if opioids have been given) and may cause undesirable dystonic reactions.

ASSESSMENT OF PHYSICAL STATUS

One must decide whether the child is 'fit' for the procedure. In the case of neonates, prematurity (see below) may present particular problems. Certain syndromes are associated with congenital malformations of the head and jaw (e.g. Treacher Collins syndrome) which may make intubation difficult or impossible.

It is very common for children undergoing simple general surgery to have concomitant congenital heart disease, which may be symptomatic or undiagnosed. The question then arises of whether there is an increased risk from anaesthesia and surgery altering cardiac shunts or giving problems with a fixed cardiac output. In most cases, knowledge of the lesion enables a safe technique to be planned. The question of antibiotic cover should always be considered in these cases, even if the surgery is trivial. Routine measurement of blood pressure is not recommended in children under 5 years but should be attempted in the sick child, especially those with renal disease, headache, and those with a family history of hypertension. No single reading should be taken as absolute but trends are important.

Cardiac murmurs

It is quite common for anaesthetists dealing with children to discover a murmur. This may be the first time the child has had a physical examination. Such murmurs are often missed by junior house staff. Most of these murmurs are 'innocent' and require no further action. If the murmur is 'pathological' it is wise to seek a cardiological opinion before surgery. Often the cardiologist can perform echocardiography on the child the same day to exclude structural anomalies.

Some guidelines may be offered to differentiate 'innocent' from 'pathological' murmurs (Table 5.1), although these are somewhat didactic.

Murmurs may also be confused with a venous hum, a continuous blowing sound heard in the neck and upper precordium. Jugular compression may alter or remove it, and its character changes with movement of the head. It disappears when the child lies down. The intensity of loudness of a murmur does not necessarily indicate its severity, as some pathological murmurs may be soft (e.g. in atrial septal defect).

There are two types of innocent murmurs.

1. A soft systolic ejection type murmur heard in the pulmonary area. It is intensified by increased cardiac output as occurs with anxiety, fever, or after exercise.

2. A vibratory type of short systolic murmur heard at the left sternal edge or sometimes the apex. Its intensity and quality vary when the child sits or changes position from side to side.

Table 5.1   Guidelines for differentiating cardiac murmurs

Innocent murmurs	Pathological murmurs
Always systolic, usually not pansystolic	Pansystolic or diastolic, may be accompanied by a thrill
Tend to diminish in volume in late systole	Associated with other cardiac symptoms or signs
No associated thrill	
Normal 2nd heart sound with normal splitting	
No other cardiac signs or symptoms	

Neurological or musculoskeletal disease may result in a greatly diminished respiratory reserve, necessitating post-operative ventilation.

Every patient should receive a full clinical pre-operative examination of the cardiovascular and respiratory system by a doctor with some experience of examining children. It is preferable if the anaesthetist who is to anaesthetize the child carries out the examination, but this is not always possible in a busy hospital. The child's urine should be tested and the temperature taken if there is any evidence of respiratory tract infection such as a runny nose. The child should be weighed in minimal clothing to enable correct calculation of dosage to be made.

PREMATURITY

In the case of children under 6 months of age, prematurity must be considered an important factor. Respiratory and cardiovascular function is affected as well as the ability to handle drugs. Even the normal full-term neonate has immature respiratory control compared with the older child or adult, and the lungs are not fully developed (see Chapter 1). Premature infants are more prone to periodic breathing and apnoea and are more likely to suffer hypoxaemia. Those whose post-conceptual age is less than 41 weeks and postnatal age less than 12 weeks are most at risk.[4] It is considered that premature infants are at increased risk of post-operative apnoea up to 44 weeks post-conceptual age,[5] but the exact post-conceptual age at which apnoea ceases to be a problem remains contentious. For this reason, many anaesthetists consider it unwise to administer opioids to this group of patients. It must be stressed, however, that preterm infants may stop breathing after any form of general anaesthesia, even when no opioids are used. Apnoea monitoring should therefore be carried out post-operatively for at least 12 h. Apnoea, if it is going to occur, usually occurs within 12 h post-operatively. Monitoring should be continued for a further 12 hours following an apnoeic spell.

Preterm infants are surfactant deficient and it is usual for them to have a degree of atelectasis until several weeks post-delivery. This may lead to post-operative pneumonia, V/Q mismatch, and intrapulmonary shunting. The resulting hypoxaemia may reinforce the tendency to apnoea or periodic breathing. In addition, many premature infants are suffering or have suffered from respiratory distress syndrome or bronchopulmonary dysplasia with consequent deterioration in lung function.

Even with a structurally normal heart, the premature baby has immature autonomic control systems. There is also a relative deficiency of pulmonary vascular smooth muscle which makes the preterm infant more prone to heart failure when left to right shunts exist, the pulmonary vascular resistance being insufficiently high.

In preterm infants, the ductus arteriosus may remain open. It is suggested that this is due to relative insensitivity to oxygen and sensitivity to prostaglandin.

Other organs may be relatively under-perfused when the duct remains widely patent, as much of the aortic flow is directed to the pulmonary artery. This may be in part responsible for the development of necrotizing enterocolitis in some premature infants.

Myocardial contractility is reduced in premature neonates and this may be exacerbated by reduced coronary flow in the shortened diastolic time when tachycardia occurs. Respiratory distress syndrome, hypoglycaemia, hypocalcaemia, hypothermia, and infection may all increase oxygen utilization and reduce myocardial oxygen supply.

NEONATAL COURSE

In small babies, events which occurred in the neonatal period, particularly the development of respiratory distress syndrome or the need for ventilation, may have profound effects on any subsequent anaesthetic. Long-term ventilation may lead to bronchopulmonary dysplasia with a requirement for increased supplementary oxygen and high ventilator pressures.

If an infant has failed to thrive, his small body mass and poor muscle formation may lead to problems with heat loss and recovery from anaesthetic agents.

FAMILY HISTORY

It is important to know if there is a family history of inherited diseases, such as epilepsy, asthma, bleeding disorders, cystic fibrosis, or sickle-cell disease and trait. Any history of untoward problems with an anaesthetic in a relative may lead one to consider the possibility of malignant hyperpyrexia, suxamethonium sensitivity, or 'halothane hepatitis'. Very often the history is nonspecific and rather unhelpful, the parents saying that a sibling 'took a long time to wake up', for example.

Certain rare syndromes which may profoundly affect the safe conduct of an anaesthetic are often well known to the members of the family who are afflicted. Careful enquiry may reveal past problems, and being forewarned, one has time to consult an authoritative text on the disease.

PREVIOUS SURGERY AND ANAESTHESIA

As with all anaesthetic practice, a detailed anaesthetic history is desirable, but is often not available, even for babies, who are frequently transferred from one hospital to another without any anaesthetic records.

RECENT RESPIRATORY TRACT INFECTION

As mentioned above, any child with signs of upper respiratory infection should have his temperature taken. He should also have his ears inspected and have a full clinical examination of the respiratory system. A febrile child or one with any lower respiratory tract signs of infection should have elective surgery cancelled for a month. The greatest difficulty arises when a child 'has just got over a cold' and has a slight dry cough, for example. It is the author's practice not to cancel elective surgery if the child is not febrile, can breathe easily, and there are no signs of active infection (throat clear, no cervical lymphadenopathy, tympanic membranes normal, and no lower respiratory tract signs). Children with large adenoids may not have a clear nasal airway even when they are well.

The greatest perceived dangers from 'colds' are that anaesthesia and surgery may lead to pneumonia or viral myocarditis.

LABORATORY INVESTIGATIONS

Routine measurement of haemoglobin level is considered unnecessary by many anaesthetists for minor procedures such as dental work, provided the child is fit and well. For procedures where bleeding is anticipated or the procedure is more major, routine investigation should include haemoglobin estimation and urinalysis.

Other investigations should only be performed if they are indicated by the disease state or treatment need. If the result will not influence management, the test should not be done. Blood can be obtained painlessly if EMLA or amethocaine cream is applied to the venepuncture site (Fig. 5.1) at least 1 h before.[6] Heel pricks can be used in babies.

CURRENT MEDICATION

It is important to know what therapy a child is already receiving, to avoid pharmacological and pharmaceutical incompatibility with the anaesthetic agents. Any history of allergy must be documented. Often such incidents are not true 'allergy', for example vomiting caused by iron or antibiotics.

PSYCHOSOCIAL ASPECTS: ESTABLISHMENT OF RAPPORT

The pre-operative visit serves two major functions. In addition to the necessary physical assessment and history taking, it allows one to build a rapport

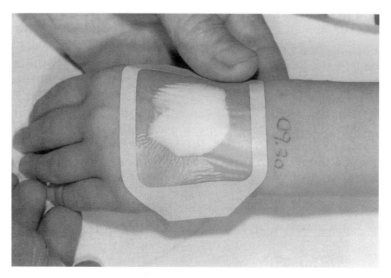

Fig. 5.1 EMLA cream.

with the child and his parents. It is clearly desirable that, to this end, they discuss the proposed anaesthetic with the doctor who is going to be there when the anaesthetic is given. If a consultant and junior will both be present, the one who has spoken to the child may then introduce the other but should continue to have the major role in conversing with the child or parent in the anaesthetic room. In the case of older children, as in adults, many anaes- thetists feel that if a good rapport is achieved and anxiety allayed, many patients do not then require premedication. It has to be said, however, that younger children do not easily come to trust a stranger, anxiety may even be heightened and premedication is often desirable, particularly if a gaseous induction is planned. The question of whether a parent should be allowed to accompany the child to the anaesthetic room often causes controversy. Most paediatric anaesthetists in the author's experience are happy to allow the parent to accompany the child provided they leave when asked to do so and do not say to the child phrases such as 'it won't hurt'. The anaesthetist must assess the parent as well on his pre-operative visit.

PREMEDICATION

Many anaesthetists consider that sedative premedication is indicated in all children, even day cases. Anticholinergic medication is rarely required with modern techniques and need not be given routinely except for small babies (who tend to be 'wet') or if ketamine is to be used. Opioids are still employed but the need for pre-operative analgesic medication can be questioned unless the child is already in pain. In that event, opioids are best given intravenously. Many anaesthetists routinely use oral benzodiazepines, chloral derivatives (e.g. triclofos or chloral hydrate), or antihistamines (e.g. promethazine or trimeprazine) for elective procedures. Oral sedation is inappropriate when gastric stasis is likely, for example following trauma or in an abdominal emergency. Less than 1.5 h may not be sufficient to allow absorption and so premedication 1.5 to 2 h pre-operatively may be preferable, especially if tablets are used.

For day cases, the advent of 'EMLA' cream has revolutionized the conduct of anaesthesia.[7] Frequently, no other medication is required and a painless intravenous induction can be performed. It is best to remove the cream a few minutes before venepuncture is attempted as the veins are less prominent immediately after the cream is wiped off. Amethocaine cream is now available for cutaneous analgesia and does not produce the vasoconstriction seen with EMLA.

BASIC ANAESTHETIC TECHNIQUE

The anaesthetic room

In the UK, children are usually anaesthetized in a room adjacent to the operating theatre. This avoids exposing the child to sights and sounds which may cause anxiety. The lighting should not be too bright and it should appear more like home than a hospital, with wall posters and with toys available to cuddle or play with. Music may help distract the child. Syringes and needles should be kept out of sight. A chair for the parent to sit on is essential as induction will frequently be performed with the child on the parent's lap. Theatre personnel must not be allowed to use the anaesthetic room as a thoroughfare during induction, and noise emanating from the theatre must be kept to a minimum.

Choice of anaesthetic technique

In this section we shall discuss the basic principles of technique which will be satisfactory for most types of general and body surface surgery. Specialized requirements are covered more fully in Chapter 8. The technique to be used is in part dictated by the condition to be treated, and therefore the surgical conditions required, and partly by the preference of the anaesthetist.

Apparatus checks

In children, deterioration can occur with frightening speed. It is therefore vital to check that everything is working properly before embarking upon the induction. Two laryngoscopes must always be available, together with suction and a range of masks and endotracheal tubes (even if intubation is not contemplated). Atropine and suxamethonium should be instantly available in case of bradycardia or laryngospasm.

Assistance

Good anaesthetic assistance is vital. The anaesthetic nurse or technician should be able to anticipate the anaesthetist's needs and have the appropriate drugs or apparatus to hand.

Induction of anaesthesia

In skilled hands intravenous induction is often the most satisfactory method for both patient and anaesthetist. If this is not possible, inhalational induction followed by intravenous drugs (e.g. muscle relaxant to facilitate intubation) is usual. However, the veins may be too small to accept a plastic cannula and then direct injection through a 27 swg hypodermic needle is feasible in an anaesthetized child (Fig. 5.2).

Once the veins have 'opened up' after a few minutes of anaesthesia a plastic cannula can be inserted or a central line placed. The most difficult age is 6 months to 2 years when the hands and wrist are chubby. Less-experienced anaesthetists, or those only occasionally caring for children, may prefer inhalational induction in all small children. The veins are often more prominent when the child is breathing an inhalational agent. Metal winged needles of the 'butterfly' type frequently cut out of the vein and cannot reliably be used throughout the procedure. Following induction, a plastic cannula should be

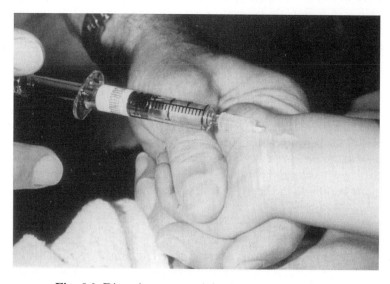

Fig. 5.2 Direct intravenous injection in a small infant.

inserted for reliable intravenous access. Blood sometimes cannot be aspirated from the needle or cannula because of low venous pressure.

Correct placement should be checked by careful administration of small quantities of saline and *never* by the use of active drug. Extravasation of thiopentone, for example, may cause skin necrosis. All drugs should be flushed in to eliminate the risk of chemical incompatibility and to ensure that the whole dose (which may be in a small volume) has been given. For a discussion of intravenous induction agents see Chapter 2.

Inhalational induction is popular for small babies and infants, even if intravenous induction is practicable. It is important to maintain continuous positive airway pressure (CPAP) on the T-piece in babies and infants. This helps to stimulate respiration in neonates and maintains a larger functional residual capacity (FRC) and decreased work of breathing in all groups where closing volume is in the tidal range (0–4 years). Volatile agents are fully discussed in Chapter 2.

Technique of inhalational induction

In all but small babies it is preferable to 'pour' the heavy vapour of an inhalational agent onto the child's face from above or across the cheek with the end of the circuit held in the anaesthetist's cupped hand. The child may be allowed to become accustomed to the apparatus and position while breathing only nitrous oxide and oxygen. Vaporizers should be turned up gradually. High concentrations, suddenly delivered, may provoke coughing, breath-holding, and laryngospasm. There is no substitute for patience. Even on a busy list, one must never be pressurized into hastening an inhalational induction. As the child becomes drowsy, the mask may be fitted to the circuit and applied snugly to the face. Jaw lift should not be applied too forcefully at this stage. No attempt should be made to insert an oral airway while the child is 'light' as this may provoke breath-holding, cough, or laryngospasm, and ruin an otherwise smooth induction. The tongue is large in small children and easily obstructs the airway. Large adenoids may compound this. A small pillow or sandbag should be placed under the shoulders and the jaw lifted forward with a finger behind the angle of the mandible. The fingers must support only bony structures. The soft tissues in the floor of the mouth are easily compressed, thereby increasing the obstruction (see Fig. 5.3). A nasopharyngeal airway may be preferable if difficulties are encountered before the jaw is fully relaxed, but bleeding from the nose or adenoids is a risk.

Intubation

Indications

In small babies, tracheal intubation is desirable, even for minor surgery, because a perfect airway may be difficult to maintain (see Table 5.2). The recently introduced laryngeal mask airway provides a valuable hands-free alternative to intubation and, in adults at least, provokes a less pronounced

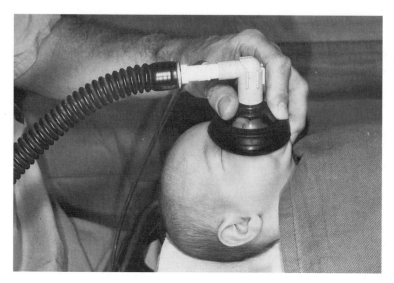

Fig. 5.3 Method of holding the face mask in a small child.

cardiovascular response. Positive pressure ventilation is, however, not recommended via the paediatric laryngeal masks. This is because the pressures generated may cause gastric distension.

In older children, the indications for intubation are similar to those in adults. In babies and small children, however, the risks of airway difficulties are higher. This is particularly true if 'peritoneal' structures such as the processus vaginalis or the anal sphincter are involved when laryngospasm may follow surgical stimulation.

Many anaesthetists feel that no patient should be allowed to breathe spontaneously for more than about an hour because of problems with absorption atelectasis, falling FRC, and hypercarbia. These are exacerbated in small children and may be worse after intubation (when the normal glottic generation of CPAP is removed) unless CPAP or IPPV is employed. Thus it is common practice to ventilate all children under about 20 kg, for anything other than brief procedures. All children under 6 months of age (or 6 kg in weight) should

Table 5.2 Indications for intubation

Age (all babies under 6 kg or 6 months of age)

Difficult airway or limited access such as ENT or head and neck surgery

Requirement for positive pressure ventilation (physical status of patient *or* type of surgery requiring muscle relaxation)

Emergency surgery (risk of regurgitation)

Prolonged procedures (exact time depends on personal preference)

be intubated, whatever the procedure, unless it is to last only a few minutes. CPAP can be applied simply by allowing the reservoir bag to become distended by partial occlusion of the open tail, but this greatly increases the resistance. For this reason IPPV is usually employed in intubated babies.

Technique of intubation

The laryngeal musculature must be fully relaxed before intubation is attempted. In babies and small infants, the laryngeal reflexes are very active; laryngospasm, bradycardia, and bronchospasm all occur very easily and with frightening speed. A controlled situation can very rapidly deteriorate into one of panic. Venous access is highly desirable before intubation is attempted in small children (under 20 kg). Children are often intubated under deep inhalational anaesthesia, but this technique is not to be recommended in neonates and small infants who frequently stop breathing before they are deeply enough anaesthetized to prevent laryngospasm. Some anaesthetists routinely give an anticholinergic drug to reduce vagal activity. Halothane provides better intubating conditions than other volatile agents. Babies and infants (under 2 years of age) are best given a muscle relaxant prior to intubation.

Awake intubation

This practice, once very popular, has declined in recent years, due to fears of intraventricular haemorrhage[8,9] and the ability of neonates to mount a considerable 'stress response'.[10] It should be reserved for moribund patients requiring resuscitation.

Apparatus

Tracheal tubes and connectors are discussed in Chapter 3. Straight blade laryngoscopes are usually used for neonates and infants, the large floppy epiglottis being lifted out of the way by the straight blade. The blade should be passed slightly into the oesophagus and then withdrawn until the larynx falls into view. The straight blade is not designed to be placed anterior to the epiglottis as are the curved (Macintosh) types, but can be used this way.

The 'difficult' airway

There are several conditions which may produce difficulty in maintaining a patent airway during anaesthesia. These are given in Table 5.3.

The difficult intubation

In adults, many ingenious ways of intubating the trachea have been devised such as fibreoptic laryngoscopy, retrograde passage of an epidural catheter, endotracheal tubes with a dirigable tip, and, of course, blind nasal intubation. All of these techniques are more difficult in children, and the more so because any one person's experience is limited. The fibreoptic broncho-

Table 5.3   Causes of a 'difficult' airway

- Craniofacial anomalies
  (e.g. Pierre Robin and Treacher Collins syndromes)
- Choanal atresia (oral intubation usually possible)
- Macroglossia (e.g. the large tongue of Down's and Beckwith's syndromes)
- Laryngo- or tracheomalacia (congenital stridor)
- Subglottic stenosis (congenital or acquired)
- Laryngeal webs
- Vascular ring (causing tracheal compression)
- Tumours (e.g. cystic hygroma)
- Nerve palsies (congenital, trauma, or surgical division of recurrent laryngeal nerve)
- Infective, e.g. croup, acute epiglottitis (see Chapter 12), quinsy (peritonsillar abscess), diphtheria
- Inhaled foreign body (all children with stridor must have this excluded)
- Trauma (to laryngeal or tracheal cartilages, facial bones; inhalation of blood etc.)
- Burns (steam and smoke inhalation acutely; scar formation later may lead to flexion of neck and limited jaw opening)

---

scopes generally available will not pass through the small endotracheal tubes used for babies, (although a 2.2 mm instrument is manufactured), and retrograde cannulation may be impossible.

A range of laryngoscope blades to suit limited mouth opening (e.g. Miller and Polio blades) with aids such as the Huffman prism are available for adults and may be of use in larger children, but for babies and infants the choice is strictly limited.

A range of straight and curved bladed laryngoscopes should be available, as one may be better than another. Some of the tubular types (e.g. Sharrard) have proved useful in this respect. Recently, it has been suggested that an endotracheal tube or introducer can be passed into the trachea via a laryngeal mask airway (see p. 56). An elective tracheostomy using ketamine or mask anaesthesia may need to be performed prior to major surgery. Local techniques are less suitable for children.

Complications of intubation are summarized in Table 5.4.

Table 5.4   Complications of intubation

- Incorrect placement (endobronchial, oesophageal)
- Obstruction (kinking, mucus, blood)
- Disconnection
- Vocal cord damage — hoarseness post-operatively
- Trauma to hypopharynx, subglottic oedema (peak incidence 1–3 years. Always check for a leak around uncuffed tubes)
- Post-extubation laryngospasm

Extubation

The endotracheal tube should be removed either when the patient is still in a state of surgical anaesthesia or awake, with reflexes returned. Even in neonates, the risk of laryngospasm is greater when the child is 'half anaesthetized', as reflex activity appears heightened. Laryngospasm is first treated by face-mask oxygen with CPAP applied via the distended bag of the circuit. If this fails, the child should be re-intubated using suxamethonium if oxygen saturation has fallen below 80 per cent. Intravenous atropine should always accompany the administration of suxamethonium in this situation.

General paediatric surgery

For body surface surgery or minor orthopaedics, inhalational techniques or propofol infusion supplemented by small doses of opioids and local anaesthetics are usually employed, with or without intubation as appropriate. Local or regional nerve blocks are being increasingly used to supplement general anaesthesia. Epidural or subarachnoid blocks may be difficult to perform without general anaesthesia but awake spinal anaesthesia for neonates[11,12] is feasible. The arms may need to be lightly bandaged together. Premedication alone may be sufficient sedation, but frequently nitrous oxide and oxygen are required to keep the child still. Regional techniques are discussed in Chapters 8 and 11 and specific techniques applicable to specialized surgery in Chapter 8.

Day care surgery

There is an increasing trend to operate on children as day cases. This brings its own problems of starvation, pre-operative assessment, and technique. A full appraisal of these problems is given in Chapter 9.

Vascular access

Vascular access, both venous and arterial, can be difficult in small or sick children. This is reviewed further below (see section 'Anaesthesia for the sick child').

Recovery from anaesthesia

It is essential that full reversal of neuromuscular blockade and return to adequate spontaneous ventilation has been achieved before the child leaves the operating theatre. Many neonates will be transferred ventilated to the intensive care unit. The child should not be sent to the recovery room in pain. This is best treated immediately in the theatre.

A fully staffed and equipped area for recovery from anaesthesia is nowadays considered essential. This should be adjacent to the theatre and should not necessitate the use of public thoroughfares or lifts. Sadly many British hospitals fall short of this ideal.

Routine oxygen therapy given until the patient is awake presents no risk from oxygen toxicity and is to be recommended for all patients. After major surgery, the need for oxygen therapy following return to the ward should be assessed by the anaesthetist and his decision written on the recovery chart.

Methods of pain relief after paediatric surgery are discussed in Chapter 11, and the pharmacology of analgesics in Chapter 2.

Routine monitoring of the airway and adequacy of respiration is ensured by the trained recovery nurse. Blood pressure measurement using non-invasive oscillometry is now routine. Urine output, wound drainage, and gastric aspirates should be recorded, together with the volumes and types of fluid administered in the operating theatre.

Fluid therapy

The child should always be presented for surgery in a state of adequate hydration. Intravenous fluids and electrolytes are usually given if the starvation period exceeds 6 h (4 h in neonates).

Venous access may be difficult in small children, particularly between the ages of 6 months and 2 years when there is much subcutaneous fat. Plastic cannulae are preferred to winged needles as they 'tissue' less often, but may be more difficult to insert. Sometimes the Seldinger technique can be used to advantage once a metal needle has been placed in the vein. Making a hole in the skin with a needle larger than the cannula to be used prevents 'burring' of the plastic on insertion. Central venous cannulation or a cut-down must be resorted to if no peripheral veins are available.

Intravenous fluids

One needs to supply the child's normal maintenance fluid requirement (Table 5.5) in addition to the operative losses, which will vary according to the size of the patient, the procedure, and the ambient temperature and humidity. Losses are best assessed on a surface-area basis, but for practical

Table 5.5   Guidelines for fluid maintenance requirements

	ml kg^{-1} h^{-1}	ml kg^{-1} 24 h^{-1}
First ten kg body weight	4	100
Next ten kg	2	50
Subsequent kg	1	20

Thus for a child weighing 27 kg, fluid requirement is $(10 \times 100) + (10 \times 50) + (7 \times 20) = 1640$ mls in 24h.

This formula is modified to maintain urine output of 2ml/kg/h.

purposes are based on a volume per kilogram calculation. Fluids used are usually 5 or 10% glucose with 0.18% or 0.225% saline (1/5 or 1/4 'normal' saline), 2.5% glucose with 0.45% saline, 0.9% saline or Ringer–Lactate (Hartmann's) solution. Care must be taken to avoid *hyperglycaemia* if glucose is given during the operative period. (Increased levels of circulating cate-cholamines may cause considerable insulin resistance.) Infants utilize three times as much water per kilogram than adults.

The kidney is less efficient in concentrating urine and the daily turnover of water is 50 per cent of the extracellular fluid volume in an infant. Various formulae are quoted for the assessment of maintenance requirements. It is important to remember that losses may be doubled during intra-abdominal or intrathoracic procedures.

Operative losses

These are commonly replaced initially with crystalloid, either glucose-saline, 0.9 per cent saline, or Hartmann's solution. Giving large quantities of crys-talloid, however, eventually results in peripheral oedema, especially if the plasma oncotic pressure is low due to haemodilution or disease. For this reason many anaesthetists prefer to use a mixture of crystalloid and colloid to replace initial operative losses. Colloids commonly employed are urea-linked or succinylated gelatin, human albumin solution (HAS), and fresh frozen plasma (FFP). FFP has the advantage that it contains clotting factors, which may be important in neonatal surgery, the immature liver being incapable of synthesis of sufficient amounts of these. There is, however, the theoretical risk of transmission of infection. This is much less likely to occur with HAS, which is pasteurized. HAS seems to offer little advantage over the gelatins for operative use in older children.

Blood may be required and is generally given in children after losses of 10–20 per cent of the circulating blood volume. Routine cases, where significant blood loss is not expected, often do not have a haemoglobin measurement made. It should, however, be done for all major cases and in all unwell children.

Anaemia

Pre-operative anaemia may need to be corrected by blood transfusion if operation is urgent or the patient is sick.

To calculate how much blood to give one can use the formula:

$$\frac{\text{(Hb required–measured Hb)}}{\text{Hb required}} \times \text{volume per kg}^* \times \text{weight of child (kg)}$$

*blood volume per kilogram according to age — see Table 5.6.

This gives the amount of whole blood to transfuse. If concentrated red cells are used, an overestimate will result. The quantity can then be reduced

Table 5.6   Variation in blood volume with age

Age	Blood volume (ml kg^{-1})
Neonate to 1 year	80–85
2 years	70
Over 3 years	60–65

according to the haematocrit of the blood to be transfused. The blood should be as fresh as possible to reduce 2,3-diphosphoglycerate depletion (see Chapter 1).

Haemoglobin level

Argument continues as to what constitutes an acceptable pre-operative haemoglobin level. In the chronically anaemic subject, adaptation to the lower quantity of haemoglobin takes place. In situations of acute blood loss, haemolysis, or severe stress, higher levels are required. A level of 10 g dl^{-1} is usually quoted as a figure to aim for pre-operatively, but 8 g dl^{-1} is probably safe if surgery cannot be delayed.

Blood transfusion

The desirability of ensuring an 'adequate' oxygen carrying capacity is obvious. Quite what constitutes 'adequate' is less obvious. The mere achievement of a particular haemoglobin level tells us little about oxygen carriage and delivery since many others factors (e.g. 2,3-diphosphoglycerate) also play a part (see Chapter 1).

Transfusion of old, stored blood is inappropriate for the severely ill. The blood used should be as fresh as possible.

Transfused blood must be warmed and (if more than 48 h old) filtered to remove micro-aggregates which may cause obstruction of pulmonary capillaries. Resuspended red cells (SAGM) are useful to restore colloid and provide haemoglobin but contain no plasma and are considered unsuitable for neonates, where FFP and vitamin K may also be required.

Administration of cold blood rapidly leads to hypothermia in small children. Low body temperature reduces citrate metabolism. Hypocalcaemia may occur, resulting in myocardial depression. For this reason it is wise to measure plasma-ionized calcium during large or rapid transfusion of whole blood, especially in small children.

For the measurement of blood loss see Chapter 4.

ANAESTHESIA FOR THE SICK CHILD

The basics of paediatric anaesthesia have been covered earlier in this chapter. Children are very resilient but in severe illness they often deteriorate with

- Air trapping may occur so nitrous oxide should be avoided.

- As low a ventilator pressure as possible should be employed with long expiratory times (to allow 'slow' alveoli to empty).

- 'Normal' PCO_2 values should not be sought. It is sufficient to ventilate the child to (or slightly above) the pre-operative value as obtained on an arterialized capillary blood gas.

- Hyperoxia should be avoided in the premature infant, oxygen saturation being maintained at 95%.

- Regional techniques (subarachnoid or epidural block) should be used whenever feasible but may be difficult in the older infant since general anaesthesia may be required to prevent movement.

Croup and epiglottitis

For a discussion of croup and epiglottitis see Chapter 12.

THE EYE

Retinopathy of prematurity (ROP)

Sometimes called retrolental fibroplasia, retinopathy of prematurity is characterized by proliferation of new retinal vessels, thrombosis, and the formation of arteriovenous anastomoses. Retinal detachment may even occur, but these abnormal processes do not occur after 44 weeks postconceptual age when vascularization of the retina is completed[6].

Although high concentrations of inspired oxygen have usually been implicated in ROP, its development is multifactorial. It has even been reported in babies given no supplementary oxygen in cyanotic heart disease[7] and in still-births[8]. There may also be some relationship to arterial PCO_2[9] and maternal diabetes. The greatest risk factor, however, is extreme prematurity.

Exposure to high oxygen tensions results in vasoconstriction of retinal vessels followed by the pathological changes described above.

Although oxygen administration resulting in hyperoxia is certainly incriminated in the development of ROP, oxygen must not be withheld if it is indicated and the infant allowed to become hypoxic. Careful monitoring by a transcutaneous oxygen electrode or blood gases is preferable since pulse oximetry cannot detect hyperoxia. An arterial PO_2 of 70–75 mmHg should be maintained. If possible, surgery should be postponed until after 44 weeks postconceptual age.

- careful monitoring is essential

- hyperoxia is dangerous to the eye at less than 44 weeks postconception but:

- hypoxia *must* be avoided. (SaO_2 values of 93–95% are acceptable). The PaO_2 should be maintained at 70–75 mmHg.

ENDOCRINE DISEASE

Diabetes mellitus

Diabetes mellitus is a common condition. The patients are almost always insulin-dependent ('juvenile' diabetes). Infants rarely manifest the disorder but it occurs in 1 in 1200 school-children. There is an association with mumps and coxsackie B4 infection as well as genetic factors. Classical symptoms of polyuria and thirst with glycosuria point to the diagnosis. Tolerance tests are rarely required if blood glucose is elevated. Ketoacidosis is a medical emergency necessitating fluid resuscitation, primarily with saline. Correction of the acidosis occurs spontaneously; bicarbonate is almost never required. Pre-operative assessment of the diabetic patient must include blood glucose and electrolytes, urine test for ketones, and state of hydration. Hartmann's solution is best avoided in diabetics, as lactate is not well tolerated.

Peri-operative management

Routine cases should be admitted the day before surgery and placed first or early on the list. Starvation should not be prolonged. If the diabetes is not well controlled, several days should be allowed for stabilization in hospital. A well-controlled diabetic can be managed by omitting breakfast and the morning insulin, post-operative control being achieved with sliding scale neutral insulin. For afternoon operations, breakfast (or the equivalent calories as a glucose infusion) should be given and long-acting insulin avoided. Five per cent glucose and insulin infused intravenously provides the best control. For all major surgery, and all emergencies this is the method of choice. The solution should contain potassium chloride 10 mmol per 500 ml of 5 per cent glucose. It is important to remember that certain plastics adsorb insulin so the dose in the bag or syringe may need to be increased above that expected from calculation of insulin requirements. One should begin insulin infusion at 0.1 units kg^{-1} h^{-1} of neutral insulin and adjust the rate according to hourly glucose oxidase strip tests. Regular laboratory estimation of electrolytes and blood sugar are required. Moderate hyperglycaemia (up to 10 mmol 1^{-1}) is permissible for urgent surgery. If ketoacidosis occurs (due to infection, for example) expert advice should be sought and the operation postponed if at all possible.

Beckwith–Wiedmann and Prader–Willi syndromes

In both these rare syndromes patients may manifest hypoglycaemia. Beckwith–Wiedmann syndrome is characterized by macroglossia, omphalocele, and gigantism. Prader–Willi patients are hypotonic and may be obese with, sometimes, overt diabetes mellitus. One should be aware of the possibility of severe hypoglycaemia occurring during anaesthesia. These children should be frequently monitored as for the diabetic patient, with glucose oxidase reagent strips both intra- and post-operatively.

Adrenal disorders

Cushings syndrome

This is rare in children. It may result from hypersecretion of cortisol by a tumour or in adrenal hyperplasia. Pituitary tumours secreting excess adrenocorticotrophic hormone (ACTH) may also result in the syndrome. Operation for removal of a tumour or adrenalectomy will require appropriate steroid cover (p. 110). Handling adrenal tumours may cause swings in blood pressure with occasional severe hypertension.

Addison's disease

Again rare, the disease is due to autoimmune adrenocortical insufficiency. It is associated with diabetes mellitus, thyroiditis, and hypoparathyroidism. Hypotension and hypokalaemia are features. Such patients receive glucocorticoid and mineralocorticoid supplements. Hydrocortisone cover is required for surgery (see p. 110). 'Adrenal crisis' may occur necessitating hydrocortisone, glucose, and saline replacement, and attention to acid base status.

Adrenogenital syndrome (congenital adrenal hyperplasia)

This is a group of autosomal recessive disorders. Absence of certain enzymes blocks various stages of the pathway of aldosterone and cortisol synthesis. The characteristics of the disease depend upon which enzyme is affected. Interruption of the feedback loop results in excessive ACTH production. This stimulates those synthetic processes which occur prior to the block, resulting in excessive androgen production. 21-hydroxylase block may lead to salt loss and adrenal crisis, 11-hydroxylase block, a step further down the pathway, produces salt retention and hypertension. Other, rarer, forms exist.

Hydrocortisone and fludrocortisone replacement is required necessitating steroid cover for surgery (see p. 110).

Thyroid disorders

Ectopic thyroid tissue may produce a thyroglossal cyst. Anaesthetic problems may result from goitres, making intubation difficult, or hyper- and hypothyroidism.

Hyperthyroidism

Hyperthyroidism may rarely occur in neonates born to mothers with a history of thyrotoxicosis. It is due to maternal thyroid-stimulating hormone crossing the placenta. The condition is transient but may produce cardiovascular signs, immobility, and fever.

Hyperthyroidism similar to that in adults occurs in childhood and 'juvenile hyperthyroidism' may undergo remission after treatment with carbimazole. Autoimmune goitres are fairly common. Most patients are euthyroid but mild hyperthyroidism (or hypothyroidism) may occur. Small thyroid nodules may be carcinomatous.

All but the most urgent surgery should be postponed if thyrotoxicosis is not controlled. Most problems are mechanical due to the goitre, with difficulty in intubation.

Hypothyroidism

Congenital and acquired forms exist. Growth retardation, macroglossia, hypotonia, umbilical hernia, and mental retardation (cretinism) are features. Centrally acting depressant drugs may produce an exaggerated response. Hypotension is likely and the stress response is poorly mounted. Hydrocortisone and thyroid hormone replacement should be given.

Steroid therapy

Many children are receiving steroids as part of their therapy, e.g. immunosuppression or asthma. Some require physiological replacement, e.g. for Addison's disease. Such patients require increased doses of steroids, particularly glucocorticoids, in times of stress. Peri-operatively this is usually given as hydrocortisone 2 mg kg^{-1}. Intravenous doses should be given until oral therapy can be recommenced. If this is likely to be delayed, the dose of hydrocortisone should gradually be reduced until it is equivalent to the previous maintenance dose.

Steroid cover should be given if the patient has received systemic steroids within the last 3 months but is unnecessary if only topical steroids have been administered.

NEUROMUSCULAR DISORDERS

Muscle diseases comprise the dystrophies, myotonias, and myopathies. Cardiovascular and respiratory problems occur and some of these muscle disorders have been cited as being associated with malignant hyperpyrexia, although the evidence for this, like strabismus, is inconclusive. Muscle relaxants must be used with great caution.

Dystrophies

Perhaps the best known and most serious is Duchenne's muscular dystrophy. It is inherited as an X-linked recessive and presents in early childhood. Most die in teenage mainly from respiratory infection. Several muscular dystrophies exist. The pelvic and shoulder girdle muscles are mostly involved in Erb's juvenile dystrophy. The facioscapulohumeral type is more slowly progressive.

Myotonias

Myotonia is a state of sustained contraction of the muscle. It is made worse by exposure to cold. The effect is in the muscle fibre and is therefore unresponsive to non-depolarizing muscle relaxants. Myotonia may be made worse by suxamethonium. These patients may be on steroid therapy and the dose will need to be increased for surgery. Two main types are recognized: the first is known as myotonia congenita and is a mild disease; dystrophia myotonica is more serious and worsens after childhood. Other systems are involved, with cataract and endocrine disease (thyroid, diabetes mellitus) and cardiac conduction anomalies being common. Despite the myotonia, the patients are weak due to loss of muscle bulk and abnormal contraction/or-not both relaxation. Relaxant drugs are therefore not indicated except for intubation.

Myopathies

There are many types. Those of most note are mentioned here:

Congenital type.

Familial periodic paralysis of which there are hyper- and hypokalaemic types. Cardiac arrhythmias may occur and pre-operative electrolyte and ECG studies are mandatory. Intra-operative potassium and blood gas measurements are advisable. If the condition is known to exist, expert help from a neurologist should be sought.

Dermatomyositis. This is manifest as a characteristic rash, proximal muscle weakness, and a vasculitis resembling polyarteritis.

Central core disease. These patients frequently manifest kyphoscoliosis or congenital dislocation of the hip (CDH). The defect is in the muscle fibre itself. There may be an association with malignant hyperpyrexia.

Myasthenia

Myasthenia gravis may present in childhood. The childhood forms may be classified as follows.

Neonatal:
(a) transient (family history; lasts a few weeks only);
(b) persistent (rare, no family history).

Juvenile:
(a) generalized, affecting all muscle groups;
(b) ocular, confined to the extra-ocular muscles.

Edrophonium ('Tensilon') may be used to aid diagnosis ($0.1-0.4$ mg kg^{-1} produces a marked improvement).

Treatment includes thymectomy and treatment with an anticholinesterase (pyridostigmine or neostigmine). Steroids are also occasionally used (extra doses will be required peri-operatively).

Muscle relaxation is rarely required peri-operatively, especially if volatile agents are employed. If non-depolarizing relaxants are used, long-acting agents should be avoided and neuromusclar function monitored with a nerve stimulator.

Myasthenia and cholinergic crises

Inadequate or no treatment results in respiratory insufficiency, due to muscle weakness. Overdosage with anticholinesterases can lead to cholinergic blockade of the neuromusclar junction with similar weakness, inability to cough, and inadequate ventilation, complicated by excessive secretion.

Central nervous system diseases

Cerebral palsy

Central nervous system (CNS) damage in utero or due to birth asphyxia or infection may lead to CNS injury. Most are spastic, some with athetoid movements, and a few have ataxia. Many also suffer epileptic seizures. Patients with cerebral palsy typically have speech defects and are mentally retarded. These children often come to surgery for major osteotomies or multi-level muscle releases to improve the disability engendered by their spasticity. The operations, usually on older children, may be long and complex.

Epilepsy

Epilepsy is common. Most children are on some form of medication (e.g. sodium valproate, phenobarbitone, or phenytoin). These drugs may significantly affect the requirement for anaesthetic drugs and their metabolism. Due to enzyme induction and chronic medication they are sometimes relatively resistant to induction of anaesthesia and higher doses than normal of pre- and post-operative sedative drugs may be required.

Plasma levels may be required post-operatively to monitor changes in requirement for anticonvulsant drugs. Enflurane may provoke convulsions in the presence of hypocarbia.

Friedreich's ataxia

These children present with ataxia, pes cavus, kyphoscoliosis, and congenital heart disease.

Riley–Day syndrome (Familial dysautonomia)

There is a defect in autonomic function with inadequate sympathetic tone and inability to cope with drug-induced vasodilation. Neonates are unable to suck and tend to aspirate. Temperature control is also affected. These children have diminished sensitivity to pain, lack of taste buds, and manifest hypotonia. Impaired sensation commonly leads to corneal ulceration. Unexplained abdominal pain may be a presenting feature. The condition is inherited as an autosomal recessive in Ashkenazy Jews.

Muscle relaxants are safe but volatile agents should be minimally employed due to cardiovascular instability.

Scoliosis

Scoliosis is relatively common but early bracing has reduced the need for operation. Correction of the curve may lead to worsening of lung function, which is frequently impaired pre-operatively. Posterior and transthoracic (anterior) approaches may be required in the same patient. The spine is usually fused with the aid of the Harrington Rod type of fixation which enables the spinal column to be straightened in a controlled manner. Distraction of the spine may lead to loss of spinal cord function and monitoring of somatosensory evoked potentials is now considered mandatory.

The anaesthetic technique should be opioid based and utilize only low concentrations of volatile agents in order not to suppress the evoked potentials. Major blood loss is usual and the surgery may take many hours. Post-operatively epidural analgesia may be administered via a catheter placed under direct vision at the end of operation.

Moebius syndrome

This condition is due to agenesis of the VI and VII cranial nerve nuclei. Micrognathia may cause difficult intubation. Aspiration pneumonia is common.

LIVER AND KIDNEY

The liver

The liver is remarkable in its functional reserve. Impairment must be severe to significantly affect the handling of most drugs.

Major problems resulting from liver disease are a tendency to severe bleeding and hypoproteinaemia. There may be a risk of contracting hepatitis and so the patient's risk status must be appreciated. Citrate metabolism may be affected and massive transfusion may lead to coagulation difficulties.

'Halothane hepatitis'

Jaundice and mildly raised hepatic enzyme levels or fulminant hepatic failure has been reported even after a single anaesthetic. The incidence in children is unknown, but probably lower than in adults.[10,11] Only 2 per cent of 701 patients quoted by Brown and Gandolfi were under 20 years of age.[11]

Kenna *et al.*[12] suggest that risk is sufficiently established to avoid halothane if other means of anaesthesia are feasible. Risk v. benefit must be assessed as halothane is easier to use and can be considered safer in the hands of inexperienced junior or the occasional paediatric anaesthetist. There are fewer airway problems such as coughing or laryngospasm than with other agents.

Kenna suggests that the diagnosis of halothane-associated liver damage can confidently be made serologically by the detection of antibody to altered liver cell membrane.[12] Antibodies, however, are only demonstrable in about 75 per cent of patients, either adult or paediatric. The diagnosis is therefore sometimes unconfirmed. There is also some doubt as to the validity of the test or the immune basis for toxicity of the agent.[11,13,14]

Other causes of jaundice must be excluded, such as sepsis, hypotension, hypoxia, drug toxicity of other kinds, malignancy, and cholestasis.

As in adults, not all causes of 'anaesthetic-associated hepatitis' develop fulminant liver failure. The only sign may be post-operative fever, perhaps prolonged nausea or a rash. Anaesthetists may not be informed of these sequelae and their significance may be missed. They may not even be documented by the house staff.

Predisposing factors

The only clear factor in children seems to be multiple exposures (maximum susceptibility within 28 days).[13]

In adults, obesity, middle age, and female gender are believed to be important. There may be a pharmacogenetic defect related to detoxification ability.[15]

The exact mechanism of halothane toxicity is unknown but the degree of biotransformation seems important. A change from the normal oxidative to reductive metabolism, free radical production, and immunological mechanisms have all been implicated. For a review, the reader is referred to Brown and Gandolfi.[11]

Multiple exposure to halothane is thought to greatly increase the risk of hepatic failure. Biotransformation is much less with the halogenated ethers (see Table 2.1). It is attractive to believe that this accounts for their lesser reported toxicity.

Enflurane has, however, also been implicated as a cause of hepatitis and cross-sensitization with halothane has been suggested,[16] but not confirmed by others.[12] Isoflurane has not so far been implicated. It is still a matter for speculation whether this is due to its low biotransformation or the possibility that enough isoflurane anaesthetics have not yet been given to reveal the problem. It is certainly a much less suitable agent for inhalation induction than halothane, even in experienced hands. The very real danger of laryngospasm may be considered to outweigh the very small risk of halothane-associated hepatitis. Enflurane appears to be the best choice for inhalation induction if halothane has been recently used, although apnoea and laryngospasm may still occur.

Overall, the safety record of anaesthetic drugs compared with other groups is enviable. Considering the millions of administrations of halothane since 1956, its safety record is truly remarkable. Any agent chosen to replace it must perform at least as well.

The kidney

The immaturity of the infant kidney has been alluded to in Chapter 1. In young babies care must be taken with fluid and electrolyte loads as the immature kidney cannot excrete large sodium, hydrogen ion, and water loads, nor can it concentrate well. Gross metabolic derangements may occur peri-operatively in the sick or premature neonate.

Polycystic kidney

There are hereditary and non-hereditary types. The infantile form is inherited by an autosomal recessive gene. The kidneys are often grossly enlarged and cystic. The condition is associated with similar cysts in the liver. Renal function is often well preserved until teenage. Survival is determined by the degree of liver and kidney damage.

Renal tract obstruction

This is commonly due to pelvi-ureteric junction obstruction or urethral valves. Hydronephrosis results, often requiring percutaneous drainage to prevent renal failure, prior to surgical relief of the obstruction.

Ectopic ureter

Ureteric anomalies are common, particularly duplex systems which may be bilateral. Obstruction and reflux with consequent hydronephrosis may occur.

Bladder exstrophy

The condition is more common in males. The endothelium of the bladder is exposed and the penis is malformed (epispadias). The pubic symphysis remains open. Surgical reconstruction may be possible but involves difficult bladder neck reconstruction and so urinary diversion is often the treatment of choice.

Wilms' tumour (nephroblastoma)

This is one of the commonest childhood malignancies. Tumour tissue frequently grows to involve the renal vein or even the inferior vena cava. Metastases may occur, most frequently to the lung. Wilms' tumour is associated with other conditions such as horseshoe kidney, ureteric duplication, renal hypoplasia, and hypospadias. Treatment is by surgery and chemotherapy or radiotherapy. The major anaesthetic problems are blood loss and diminished renal function (tumours rarely occur bilaterally). Intra-operative hypertension may occur when the tumour is handled. It is wise to have a large intravenous cannula above and below the operative site so as to be able to cope with inferior vena cava obstruction during surgery. (see also p. 151).

Hypospadias

This is a common anomaly. The urethra opens onto the ventral surface of the penis. Surgical correction is required in severe cases. Caudal block is particularly suited to such operations.

Renal failure

Renal failure can be divided into acute and chronic forms.

Acute renal failure (ARF).   The usual features are oliguria with electrolyte imbalance. The causes of ARF are conventionally grouped thus:

- *pre-renal*, e.g. hypovolaemia from any cause; hypotension due to sepsis or drugs; diuretic therapy in heart failure;
- *renal*, e.g. acute tubular necrosis (ATN) (ischaemic or toxic); sepsis; acute glomerulonephritis; haemolytic-uraemic syndrome;
- *post-renal*, e.g. ureteric or urethral obstruction with hydronephrosis.

Meticulous attention to fluid balance and the preservation of urine output (with diuretics if indicated) is required. The prognosis is good, particularly from a pre-renal cause.

Chronic renal failure.   Such cases are rare, about 100 per year in Britain. Anorexia and poor nutrition are common. Many of these children will be receiving haemodialysis and awaiting transplantation. Such children may require surgery for creation of arterio-venous fistulae and coincidental surgical conditions e.g. appendicitis. Anaesthesia for *any* surgery in this group must follow the principles outlined below.

Anaesthesia for renal transplantation

One must consider the following:

- the effect of anaesthetic drugs on existing renal function: drug excretion, changes in protein binding etc.; lower albumin concentrations may affect toxicity of local anaesthetics due to increase in the unbound fraction.
- timing of operation in relation to dialysis;
- concomitant systemic disease (e.g. anaemia, heart failure, hypertension, coagulopathy and infection, particularly hepatitis).

Minimal pre-operative investigations are:

Haemoglobin (8 g dl^{-1} acceptable);

Urea and electrolytes including calcium and phosphate;
Plasma proteins;
Coagulation status;
ECG.

Anaesthetic technique   Thiopentone or propofol with low-dose opioid, atracurium or vecuronium, volatile agent and regional block supplementation is the method of choice. Drugs which are primarily renally excreted must be avoided (e.g. pancuronium). Enflurane may be associated with worsening of pre-existing renal disease. Halothane or isoflurane appear safe.

Narcotics seem to be more potent in patients with chronic renal failure. This may be due to easier passage of the blood–brain barrier in the uraemic state. Small incremental intravenous doses should therefore be given to assess the effect. Post-operative analgesia can be provided by low dose opioid or epidural infusion of bupivacaine. Great attention must be paid to circulating volume in the peri-operative period. Following dialysis, relative hypovolaemia may be present, necessitating a *small* fluid load at induction. Due to the frequent presence of hypertension, vasopressors are best avoided and epidural blockade should be instituted incrementally through a catheter to minimize changes in blood pressure.

Blood transfusion has been avoided by many clinicians due to fear of provoking an antibody response. Blood may need to be given, however, if the haemoglobin is below 8 g dl^{-1}.

CONNECTIVE TISSUE AND STORAGE DISORDERS

Connective tissue disorders

Marfan's syndrome
Marfan patients are characteristically tall and thin with spider-like fingers (arachnodactyly).

Spinal deformity occurs frequently, as does pectus excavatum, recurrent joint dislocation, dislocation of the lens of the eye, and aortic regurgitation. Aortic aneurysm may occur. The condition is inherited by an autosomal dominant gene. The main anaesthetic problems are cardiovascular.

Osteogenesis imperfecta
The connective tissue disorder is not confined to bones but is widespread throughout the body. The sclera may appear blue. Brittle bones, deafness, and a tendency to joint subluxation are constant features. The osteoblasts are abnormal and fractures easily occur. Platelet function may be abnormal.[17] Special care is needed when positioning the patient. Intubation may be hazardous in the presence of loose or carious teeth to which these children are prone.

Ehlers–Danlos syndrome

Collagen deficiency in this rare syndrome results in recurrent dislocation. The major anaesthetic problem is related to fragility of superficial veins which makes vascular access difficult, and the patients are prone to bleeding and bruising. The condition is associated with diaphragmatic and inguinal hernia. Dissecting aortic aneurysm may also occur.

Homocystinuria

This is due to deficiency of the enzyme cystathionine synthetase. The child resembles one with Marfan's syndrome but mental retardation is common. Intravascular thrombosis, arterial dissections, and hypoglycaemia may complicate anaesthesia and surgery.

Storage disorders

Several different types of genetically determined enzyme defects result in a variety of syndromes. Mucopolysaccharide or lipid pathways may be affected.

Mucopolysaccharidoses

Hurler's syndrome   Mental retardation and corneal opacity are regular features. Joint stiffness and cardiac failure occur after infancy. Most do not achieve teenage and die from coronary insufficiency, heart failure, and valve lesions, together with chest infection. They have a large tongue and poor neck mobility which may make intubation difficult. The condition is associated with inguinal and umbilical hernias which is the usual reason for presentation to the anaesthetist.

Morquio's syndrome   The main features are kyphoscoliosis which may be severe, odontoid hypoplasia, corneal opacity, and aortic regurgitation. These children are of normal intelligence.

General muscle weakness may lead to ventilatory problems. Atlanto-occipital subluxation and odontoid fracture have been reported. Great care must therefore be taken with positioning. The neck must be held in the neutral position during anaesthesia and most particularly at intubation.

Gargoylism (Hunter's syndrome)   This is very similar to Hurler's syndrome.

Lipid storage disorders

The features of these conditions are pancytopenia, hepatosplenomegaly, and failure to thrive. Death usually occurs before teenage.

Glycogen storage diseases

These include Von Gierke's disease, Pompe's disease, and others. The usual reason for anaesthesia is for liver biopsy. Von Gierke's patients are the most common of this rare group. They are prone to hypoglycaemia and lactic acidosis.

BLOOD DISORDERS

Sometimes a familial problem is identified at the pre-operative visit such as haemophilia, Christmas disease, or thalassaemia. Occasionally an inherited condition may be suspected but require confirmation, for example sickle-cell trait. The most common haematological problem for anaesthetists, however, is anaemia from whatever cause.

Anaemia

For elective surgery, many anaesthetists would not accept a child for anaesthesia if the haemoglobin level was below 10 g dl^{-1}. This ensures more than adequate oxygen-carrying capacity under normal circumstances. Individual surgical requirements and concurrent medical condition (such as renal failure or chronic blood loss) must be taken into account. In most cases chronic anaemia is accompanied by an increase in 2,3-diphosphoglycerate (2,3-DPG) which aids oxygen delivery (see Chapter 1). The normal fall in haemoglobin levels in infancy is associated with a left to right shift of the dissociation curve and a rise in 2,3-DPG levels. Thus the high neonatal haemoglobin falls to about 10 g dl^{-1} at 3 months before it begins to rise again. Interestingly, 2,3-DPG levels do not rise much in chronic renal failure[18] but oxygen delivery appears to be adequate, even with haemoglobins below 8 g dl^{-1}.

Causes of anaemia

- Blood loss: this includes sampling for investigation, which may be significant in small babies, haemorrhagic disease, hiatus hernia, Meckel's diverticulum.
- Haemolysis: hereditary spherocytosis, rhesus or ABO incompatibility, autoimmune disease, thalassaemia, sickle-cell disease, and glucose-6-phosphate dehydrogenase (G6PD) deficiency.
- Iron or folate deficiency.
- Bone marrow depression: aplastic anaemias, leukaemia, cytotoxic therapy.
- Chronic renal disease.

Sickle-cell disease

This is usually found in individuals of negro origin and is inherited as an autosomal recessive. The disease is caused by the presence of a haemoglobin variant, HbS, in the red cell. HbS differs from HbA by having valine substituted for glutamic acid in the beta-chain. The HbS chains polymerize and precipitate at low oxygen tensions which causes distortion of the red cell (sickling). The red cells are less deformable in the capillary, and blood viscosity is increased. Sludging occurs with a tendency to thrombosis and infarcts, particularly in the spleen. Individuals may possess sickle cell *trait* (HbS/HbA) or manifest the *disease* (HbS/HbS) depending on whether they are hetero- or homozygous. Electrophoresis will determine the percentage of HbS present. Homozygotes may possess up to 20 per cent fetal haemoglobin (HbF). So-called sickle cell thalassaemia (HbS/HbF) manifests more HbF (up to 30 per cent) and is a less severe condition.

A sickle *crisis* occurs when large numbers of red cells sickle due to hypoxia, acidosis, and capillary stasis, and is worsened by low temperatures. Sodium bicarbonate was once favoured routinely during anaesthesia but haemodilution is now preferred. A haematocrit of 0.30 is considered ideal to maximize blood flow in the capillary. Surgery can be safely undertaken with a haemoglobin of 8 g dl^{-1}.

Supplementary oxygen during anaesthesia and the recovery phase (and possibly for 24 h after major surgery) is essential as is meticulous airway care and avoidance of respiratory depression.

Thalassaemia

Thalassaemia is an inherited condition which results from underproduction of either α- or β-globin chains due to gene mutation. In normal adult haemoglobin the α and β chains are present in equal numbers. In α-thalassaemia there is a marked decrease or even an absence of α chains. A similar situation with β-chains gives rise to β thalassaemia.

This imbalance in globin chains leads to reduced haemoglobin synthesis with a microcytic, hypochromic anaemia. The most severe forms are rare but minor degrees of thalassaemia are very common. The severity of the anaemia is dependent upon whether the individual is hetero- or homozygous.

α-thalassaemia most commonly occurs in those of African, Malaysian, or Indo-Chinese extraction. In β-thalassaemia, more frequently found in those of African or Mediterranean origin (but also Indian and Chinese), there is usually an increase in γ- and δ-globin chains, resulting in increased production of fetal haemoglobin (HbF) and HbA2. Heterozygotes with β-thalassaemia are usually asymptomatic. The homozygous form is more severe. If *no* β-globin is produced the condition is called β-thalassaemia major, which is manifest as a severe microcytic anaemia.

Complications of thalassaemia are haemosiderosis, splenomegaly, endocrine abnormalities, including diabetes and delayed puberty. Cardiac haemosiderosis results in dilatation of the heart and dysrhythmia, most commonly supraventricular tachycardia.

These children require frequent blood transfusion and splenectomy may be required.

Bleeding disorders

Haemophilia

Classic haemophilia or haemophilia A is an X-linked recessive disorder which results in low levels of factor VIII. Because of its X-linked inheritance it only occurs in males. Carrier females are not obvious clinically. Spontaneous haemorrhage does not occur until factor VIII levels are less than 5 per cent. Bleeding following mild trauma occurs with levels of around 5–10 per cent of normal. Treatment is with cryoprecipitate which contains large quantities of factor VIII. A number of haemophiliacs have been infected with human immunodeficiency virus (HIV) due to the use of cryoprecipitate manufactured from plasma obtained abroad. These preparations are no longer used and the cryoprecipitate currently available carries negligible risk.

Christmas disease

Christmas disease is clinically identical to haemophilia A but is due to deficiency of factor IX. Inheritance is again X-linked. Treatment is with factor IX concentrate.

Von Willebrand's disease This disorder affects both males and females although clinically the pattern of bleeding differs from haemophilia in that bleeding into joints is rare. Decreased factor VIII levels are demonstrable but these patients also have a disorder of capillary and platelet function, manifest by increased bleeding time. Treatment is with cryoprecipitate

Platelet disorder Thrombocytopenia is a more usual cause of problems than platelet dysfunction. Low platelet count may be due to:

- idiopathic and familial thrombocytopenia;
- disseminated intravascular coagulation (DIC);
- leukaemias;
- Marrow aplasia due to, for example, drugs or radiation.

Treatment is by platelet transfusion when bleeding occurs or prophylactically. Children with idiopathic thrombocytopenic purpura (ITP) are often taking steroids and will require cover for operation (p. 110).

IMPORTANT CHROMOSOMAL DISORDERS

Down's syndrome (Trisomy 21: mongolism)

The features are the classical mongoloid facies, prominent transverse palmar crease, and mental retardation. Heart disease is common, particularly coarctation of the aorta and septal defects. Increased maternal age (over 40) is a definite predisposing factor. They often present for routine surgical procedures and care must be taken to assess cardiovascular status. The tongue may be rather large and make intubation less easy although it is rarely particularly difficult.

Turner's syndrome (genotype XO)

Turner's syndrome is manifested by females of short stature and failure of ovarian maturation with consequent lack of pubertal changes and infertility. Coarctation is common.

Noonan's syndrome

These children are similar in appearance to those with Turner's syndrome but chromosome studies reveal a normal karyotype. Mental retardation and congenital valvular cardiac lesions are common. Pectus excavatum and micrognathia may lead to respiratory difficulties.

CONDITIONS LEADING TO DIFFICULTY WITH INTUBATION

Several conditions may lead to airway problems and sometimes extremely difficult intubation. Micrognathia is particularly apparent in Treacher Collins syndrome, (1st branchial arch syndrome), Pierre Robin syndrome, and Goldenhar Syndrome (1st and 2nd branchial arch syndrome). Most of these syndromes are also associated with other anomalies such as congenital heart disease, cleft lip and palate.

The Pierre Robin syndrome[19,20] consists of severe micrognathia, a cleft palate, and possible epiglottic dysplasia. Unless the child is nursed prone, the tongue may become wedged in the cleft palate, causing respiratory obstruction. These children are usually of normal intelligence. A special frame is available to allow easy nursing care while maintaining the infant prone. The tongue may be anastomosed to the lower lip to prevent obstruction while the infant waits for cleft palate repair, although this is now undertaken in many centres at an earlier age than previously. The Robin anomalad

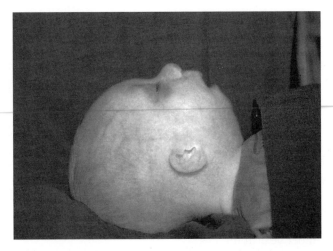

Fig. 6.1 Child with Pierre Robin syndrome showing micrognathia.

may also be seen as part of other syndromes. (Stickler; De Lange). The Treacher Collins syndrome[21] consists of micrognathia, maxillary dysplasia, abnormal ears and eyes, and sometimes a cleft palate. A family history is frequently apparent. Conductive deafness is common. The laryngeal inlet may be small, compounding difficulties with intubation. Mental retardation is not a feature.

Other conditions which may present the anaesthetist with a difficult airway include children with Moebius's syndrome who may have micrognathia, Klippel–Feil syndrome, because of limited movement of the cervical spine, and joint disorders such as juvenile rheumatoid arthritis (Still's disease) and arthogryposis multiplex. Children with storage disorders, such as Hurler's syndrome, have a short neck, large tongue, and inelastic tissues which may make laryngoscopy difficult.

Oral and pharyngeal tumours and cleft palate may cause problems in visualization of the larynx or passage of the endotracheal tube.

CONDITIONS WHERE VENTILATORY DIFFICULTIES MAY BE ENCOUNTERED

These include myotonia congenita, the muscular dystrophies, cystic fibrosis, prune belly syndrome (due to weak or absent abdominal muscles), severe scoliosis, particularly following operative correction, and children with central hypoventilation syndrome (Ondine's curse) or adenotonsillar hypertrophy causing sleep apnoea.

MALIGNANT HYPERPYREXIA (MH)

This condition is rare but when it occurs prompt treatment is required to prevent a fatal outcome. It is associated with the use of certain 'trigger' agents such as suxamethonium, and halogenated hydrocarbon anaesthetics, most commonly halothane. Certain syndromes may predispose to the condition such as Duchenne muscular dystrophy, central core disease, congenital scoliosis, osteogenesis imperfecta, and strabismus, although the latter has recently been questioned. Stress alone may precipitate MH.

MH is a familial condition with autosomal dominant inheritance. The risk of producing an affected child is 50 per cent. The reported incidence is about 1 in 15 000 children (1:10 000 in adults). MH is more frequent in females. It affects all races. It most commonly occurs between the ages of 10 and 30 years and is very rare under 5 years of age. The mortality is now 2–3 per cent (about 1 death per year in the UK).

It is impossible to clinically identify an MH susceptible patient pre-operatively but a family history of MH or an unexpected death during anaesthesia may lead to investigation of the family. *A previous history of uneventful anaesthesia does not exclude MH.* The condition seems to be more common during minor surgical procedures. Post-operative fever following a completely uneventful anaesthetic is unlikely to be due to MH. Such cases are no longer screened by muscle biopsy (see below).

Mortality may be as high as 50 per cent. The pathological basis of the disorder is sustained skeletal muscle contraction due either to sustained calcium release or failure of re-uptake by the sarcoplasmic reticulum. A similar condition can be induced in Pietrain pigs, in which there has been much experimental study. The diagnosis is essentially clinical. Signs of MH are:

- tachycardia or other dysrhythmia;
- tachypnoea (if breathing spontaneously);
- high oxygen consumption;
- hypercarbia;
- rise of core temperature — over a few minutes to 40 °C or more (sometimes the hyperthermia has a slower onset);
- metabolic and respiratory acidosis;
- hyperkalaemia;
- muscle spasm (particularly masseter spasm following suxamethonium);
- elevated CPK (serum creatine phosphokinase).

In addition cyanosis or mottling, hyper or hypotension, myoglobinuria, and disseminated intravascular coagulation may occur. The serum calcium may be high or low, providing little diagnostic help. Blood gas analysis and serum potassium estimation should be performed if unexplained tachycardia, tachypnoea, or hyperpyrexia occur. Masseter spasm occurs in about 1 per cent of children given suxamethonium.[22]

Laboratory investigation

A family history of anaesthetic problems, suggestive of MH, particularly if there has been a death, will usually lead to investigation of the family. Creatine phosphokinase (CPK) estimations in blood from the resting subject may be elevated but there are many causes of a raised CPK so that this test in itself is not diagnostic. Muscle biopsy is the currently preferred test in the UK. Patients can be referred to a centre specializing in the diagnosis of MH (e.g. in the UK, the University Department of Anaesthesia in Leeds). A family history of anaesthetic-related problems should lead to an attempt to procure the hospital notes of the patient concerned. If operation on an individual suspected of being at risk from MH cannot be delayed to allow investigation, an anaesthetic which avoids known triggering agents must be given. A 'halothane-free' anaesthetic machine must be used, avoiding rubber hoses which may have vapour dissolved in the rubber. Disposable plastic circuits are now widely available.

Screening for MH susceptibility

About 100 cases annually are referred to the Leeds MH Investigation Unit of which about 60 are screened. Of those, approximately half are found to be MH susceptible. Only muscle biopsy can provide a definitive diagnosis. Screening starts with the proband (the patient who has suffered the reaction) if possible, but if that patient has died or is aged less than 10 years the parents are screened.

In the UK patients aged less than 10 years are not screened due to problems in interpreting the results in immature muscle and because the 1–2 g of muscle required for the test is regarded as a significant amount in young children. Also, the length of the individual specimens is important.

Young children of an MH-susceptible parent are treated as potentially MH susceptible until they are old enough to be screened (Halsall, P. J., personal communication).

The test used is the *in-vitro contracture test* and is performed on a *fresh* muscle biopsy, which therefore must be obtained at the investigation centre. Small strips of muscle are exposed to halothane and caffeine. Normal muscle relaxes on exposure to halothane but MH muscle contracts; caffeine stimulates all muscle but MH muscle reacts at much lower concentrations.

Drugs which are safe to use in patients at risk include:

atracurium	metoclopramide
atropine	nitrous oxide
benzodiazepines	ANY local anaesthetic without
droperidol	vasoconstrictor
glycopyrronium	
propofol	
thiopentone	
any analgesic	
vecuronium	
neostigmine	

In the past, morphine and nitrous oxide have been implicated as trigger agents but are now considered safe. (Halsall, P.J. personal communication). Careful monitoring of the ECG, end-tidal CO_2, core temperature, and blood pressure are essential. An arterial line is highly desirable for beat-by-beat monitoring and the facility of frequent blood gas estimations.

Dantrolene

At risk patients may be pretreated with 5 mg kg^{-1} dantrolene, a skeletal muscle relaxant which probably works by indirectly limiting calcium release. This cannot be done if the anaesthetic is being given for muscle biopsy.

Treatment of established MH[23]

Intra-operative diagnosis is a *clinical* one and relies on a high index of suspicion. Treatment must be immediate upon making the diagnosis. The following plan should be followed.

- Withdraw all possible trigger agents.
- Stop surgery as soon as possible to reduce stress and shorten the duration of anaesthesia.
- Convert to oxygen (plus nitrous oxide if O_2 tension adequate)/narcotic relaxant technique using plastic circuits and an anaesthetic machine purged of volatile agents. Hyperventilation.
- Blood gas analysis and potassium estimation.
- Active cooling (e.g. peritoneal, gastric, and bladder lavage. SURFACE COOLING MAY INCREASE CORE TEMPERATURE). Leave urinary catheter *in situ* if possible.
- Intravenous dantrolene (1 mg kg^{-1} increments repeated as necessary each 10 min, until fever declines and acidosis reverses. Maximum cumulative

Table 6.1　*(Continued)*

3. Storage disorders

Condition	Relevance
Mucopolysaccharidoses 　Hurler's syndrome	Mental retardation. Clouding of the cornea Respiratory infection common. Cardiac failure Inguinal hernia Large tongue and short neck (DIFFICULT INTUBATION) Die young (10 years)
Hunter's syndrome (gargoylism)	Similar to Hurler's but less severe Mental retardation. Large tongue Cardiac disease (DIFFICULT INTUBATION)
Morquio's syndrome	Kyphoscoliosis, heart disease (aortic reflux) Possibility of odontoid fracture or atlanto-occipital subluxation. Extreme care required when positioning
Glycogen storage diseases 　Von Gierke's disease (Type 1)	Commonest type. Renal and hepatic insufficiency. PRONE TO HYPOGLYCAEMIA. Avoid lactate (Hartmann's solution)
Pompe's disease (Type 2)	Hypotonia. Large tongue. DIFFICULT AIRWAY. Cardiac failure. Early death (2 years)
Forbes' disease (Type 3)	Mild disorder. No particular anaesthetic problems. Similar to Type 1
Andersen's disease (Type 4)	Portal hypertension with cirrhosis; ascites, oesophageal varices Bleeding problems

4. Endocrine disorders

Condition	Relevance
Beckwith–Wiedemann syndrome	Large tongue, omphalocele (exomphalos) *HYPOGLYCAEMIA* DIFFICULT AIRWAY
Prader–Willi syndrome	Mental retardation. Short stature Hypotonia. *Obese.* May be diabetic DIFFICULT VENOUS ACCESS

Table 6.1   (*Continued*)

4. Endocrine disorders (Continued)

Condition	Relevance
Thyroid goitre	Rarely a problem in childhood Ensure patient is euthyroid before surgery DIFFICULT AIRWAY Tracheal compression may occur

5. Other conditions

Condition	Relevance
Asthma	Bronchospasm. Hypoxia. Atopy
Cystic fibrosis	Meconium ileus Poor lung function. Copious secretions Bronchiectasis. Broad spectrum antibiotic cover for surgery. Liver problems, oesophageal varices. Diabetes. May require portocaval shunt or injection of varices
Haemophilia Von Willebrands disease Christmas disease	Bleeding
Klippel–Feil syndrome	Cleft palate Fused cervical vertebrae (occasionally hemivertebra). Webbed neck. Deaf Heart disease. Mentally retarded. Scoliosis DIFFICULT INTUBATION
Juvenile rheumatoid	Polyarthritis Uveitis (may be blind) Pericarditis, rashes, nephritis. IF JAW OR NECK INVOLVED, MAY BE AIRWAY DIFFICULTIES
Down's syndrome (Trisomy 21)	Mental retardation Heart disease
Turner's syndrome	Short. Webbed neck Coarctation common
Noonan's syndrome	Heart disease. Micrognathia

REFERENCES

1. Morrison, J. E. Jr (1994). Chicken pox: an operating room problem? *Paediatric Anaesthesia*, **4**, 65.
2. Sandström, K. and Nilsson, K. (1995). Whooping cough and anaesthesia. *Paediatric anaesthesia*, **5**, 76.
3. Northway, W. H., Rason, R. C., and Porter, D. Y. (1967). Pulmonary disease following respiratory therapy of hyaline membrane disease. New England Journal of Medicine, **276**, 357.
4. Miller, R. W., Woo, P., Kellman, R. K. *et al.* (1987). Tracheobronchial abnormalities in infants with bronchopulmonary dysplasia. *Journal of Pediatrics*, **111**, 779.
5. Werthammer, J. Brown, E. F., Neff, R. K. *et al.* (1982). Sudden infant death syndrome in infants with bronchopulmonary dysplasia. *Pediatrics*, **69**, 301.
6. Quin, G. E., Betts, E. K., Diamond, G. R. *et al.* (1981). Neonatal age (human) at retinal maturation. *Anesthesiology*, **55**, S, 326.
7. Kalina, R. E., Hodson, W. A., and Morgan, B. C. (1972). Retrolental fibroplasia in a cyanotic infant. *Pediatrics*, **50**, 765.
8. Adamkin, D. H., Shott, R. J., Cook, L. N. *et al.* (1977). Non-hyperoxic retrolental fibroplasia. *Pediatrics*, **60**, 828–830.
9. Wolbarsht, M. L., George, G. S., Kylstia, J. *et al.* (1982). Does carbon dioxide play a role in retrolental fibroplasia? *Pediatrics*, **70**, 500.
10. Williams, N. (1986). *Halothane and the liver — the problem revisited.* Bristol Royal Infirmary.
11. Brown, B. R. Jr and Gandolfi, A. J. (1987). Adverse effects of volatile anaesthetics. *British Journal of Anaesthesia*, **59**, 14.
12. Kenna, J. G., Neuberger, V., and Mieli-Vergant, G. (1986). Halothane hepatitis in children. *British Medical Journal*, **294**, 1209.
13. Neuberger, J. and Williams, R. (1984). Halothane anaesthesia and liver damage. *British Medical Journal*, **289**, 1136.
14. Dienstage, J. L. (1980). Halothane hepatitis — allergy or idiosyncrasy. *New England Journal of Medicine*, **303**, 102.
15. Farrell, G., Prendergast, D., and Murray, M. (1985). Halothane hepatitis — detection of a constitutional susceptibility factor. *New England Journal of Medicine*, **313**, 1310.
16. Lewis, J. H. *et al.* (1983). Enflurane hepatotoxicity — a clinicopathologic study of 24 cases. *Annals of Internal Medicine*, **98**, 984.
17. Stehling, L. (1978). Anesthesia for children requiring orthopaedic surgery. *Anesthesiology Review*, **5**, 19.
18. Smith, R. M. and Strieder, D. J. (1976). Variable oxygen affinity of hemoglobin in children with uremic anemia. American Society of Anesthesiologists, San Francisco, October 1976. Quoted in *Anesthesia for infants and small children* (ed. R. M. Smith). Mosby (1980).
19. Robin, P. (1923). Backward lowering of the root of the tongue causing respiratory disturbances. *Bulletin de l'Académie Nationale de Médecine*, **89**, 37.
20. Robin, P. (1929). De la physiologique de la tétée au sein et de la forme que doit avoir tétine du bibeion. *Bulletin de la Société de Pédiatrie, Paris*, **27**, 55.
21. Treacher, J. and Collins, E. (1900). Case with symmetrical congenital notches of the outer part of each lower lid and defective development of the malar bones. *Transactions of the Ophthalmological Society, UK*, **20**, 190.

22. Lynn, A. M. (1989). Unusual conditions in paediatric anaesthesia. In *Textbook of paediatric anaesthetic practice* (ed. E. Sumner and D. Hatch) p. 529. Baillière Tindall, London.

23. Friesen, C. M., Brodsky, V. B., and Dillingham, M. E. (1979). Successful use of dantrolene sodium in human malignant hyperthermia syndrome. *Canadian Anaesthetists' Society Journal*, **26**, 319.

24. Lerman, J. *et al.* (1988). Pharmacokinetics of intravenous dantrolene in malignant hyperthermia susceptible paediatric patients. *Anesthesia and Analgesia*, **67**, (Suppl.), 133.

7

Anaesthesia for cardiac surgery

S. N. C. Bolsin and C. R. Monk

INTRODUCTION

The incidence of congenital heart disease (CHD) in the UK remains constant at 7 per 1000 live births. With a birth rate of 600 000 per annum, the number of children born with congenital heart disease will be 4000 per year. Untreated, one third of children would die within the first month, and a further third within the first year of life. The commonest associated abnormality is Down's syndrome. Deletion of a locus on chromosome 22 (22q deletion) is associated with truncus arteriosus.

CLASSIFICATION

Effective anaesthetic management of children for cardiac surgery requires an understanding of the pathophysiology of the underlying condition. These conditions can be classified into basic functional groups according to the presence or absence of central cyanosis. The presence of cyanosis indicates reduced pulmonary blood flow or right-to-left shunting as in tetralogy of Fallot, pulmonary stenosis or pulmonary atresia with ventricular or atrial septal defect (VSD or ASD), total anomalous pulmonary venous drainage (TAPVD), and tricuspid atresia. The exception is transposition of the great arteries (TGA) which has cyanosis with a high pulmonary blood flow. Absence of cyanosis in congenital heart disease implies either left-to-right shunting as in VSD, ASD, patent ductus arteriosus (PDA), and truncus arteriosus, or obstructive lesions such as aortic stenosis or coarctation of the aorta.

PHYSIOLOGY OF INTRACARDIAC SHUNTING

Right-to-left shunt

Right-to-left shunting results in decreased pulmonary and increased systemic blood flows, cyanosis, left ventricular volume overload and subsequent

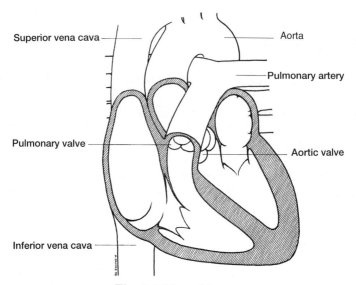

Superior vena cava

Aorta

Pulmonary artery

Pulmonary valve

Aortic valve

Inferior vena cava

Fig. 7.1 Normal heart.

failure. The reduced pulmonary blood flow produces cyanosis and metabolic acidosis, which will maintain patency of the ductus arteriosus in neonatal life. If a patent ductus is closing in infancy, patency may be maintained by an infusion of prostaglandin E_1 (0.05–0.1 μg kg^{-1} min^{-1}). This may produce apnoeic episodes and necessitate intubation and ventilation of the lungs. Further problems associated with prolonged right-to-left shunting include polycythaemia, secondary to chronic hypoxia, disorders of both platelets and clotting factors, increased risk of thrombosis, and increases in blood viscosity. These features have important anaesthetic implications.

The gaseous induction of anaesthesia is slower than expected because the partial pressure of anaesthetic gas or vapour perfusing the brain is less than the alveolar pressure due to the dilution effect of the blood by-passing the lungs. Hyperventilation can partially compensate for this effect by increasing the rate of equilibration between the inspired and alveolar gas concentrations. An intravenous induction is quicker due to some of the systemic venous blood by-passing the pulmonary circulation, causing a rapid rise in brain concentration and an apparent increased sensitivity to intravenous induction agents. The delivery of oxygen depends upon the cardiac output and the total oxygen content. Oxygenation is dependent on an adequate pulmonary blood flow (Qp) which is determined by the ratio of the pulmonary and systemic vascular resistances; thus, a relative decrease in pulmonary vascular resistance improves Qp and the oxygen content of the systemic blood.

Decreases in the cardiac output reduce oxygen delivery, causing tissue hypoxia and metabolic acidosis, thus inducing myocardial depression, with peripheral vasodilation further impairing pulmonary blood flow. Treatment is tracheal intubation, hyperventilation with 100 per cent oxygen, fluid administration (2–4 ml kg^{-1} of crystalloid or colloid), and sodium bicarbonate (1 mmol kg^{-1}). If there is a dynamic component to the right ventricular outflow tract obstruction by a muscular infundibular ring (as in tetralogy of Fallot), this is exacerbated by sympathetic stimulation producing spasm. The impaired pulmonary blood flow and hypotension is treated as above but added fentanyl (2–5 μg kg^{-1}), halothane (1.5 per cent), and, if needed, propranolol (up to 0.2 mg kg^{-1}) can be used to relax the infundibular spasm.

Palliative systemic-pulmonary connections are made in patients with poor pulmonary blood flow to improve pulmonary circulation and oxygenation. They are therefore dependent upon an adequate systemic pressure. Vasodilation and hypotension should be avoided as this will decrease shunt flow and impair oxygen delivery.

Left-to-right shunt

Left-to-right shunting results in excessive pulmonary blood flow, pulmonary hypertension, and impaired pulmonary compliance. Heart failure is caused by volume overload of the left ventricle, but the presentation is the same as for obstructive causes of heart failure in infancy, such as aortic stenosis and coarctation of the aorta.

The standard medical treatment is diuretics and digoxin, with angiotensin-converting enzyme (ACE) inhibitors now being used in severe cases. Commonly associated problems are hypokalaemia and hypovolaemia from diuretic therapy, hypoxia from pulmonary oedema with tachypnoea and eventually hypercarbia. Pulmonary compliance is decreased along with gas exchange.

In neonates, other complications include hypoglycaemia, hypocalcaemia, anaemia (sometimes iatrogenic from repeated blood testing), reduced temperature regulation, and occasionally retrolental fibroplasia from excessive oxygen therapy. There are also important anaesthetic considerations.

The gaseous induction is quicker than expected because the partial pressure of blood reaching the brain rises rapidly. This is due to the admixture of systemic blood, with a high partial pressure of vapour, to the pulmonary blood maintaining the alveolar concentration. Recirculation of intravenously administered drugs in the pulmonary circulation decreases the fraction of drug reaching the brain. This relative insensitivity requires caution or an excessive total dose of induction agent can be given.

Oxygen delivery depends on systemic blood flow, which is determined by the ratio between the pulmonary and systemic vascular resistances. Moderate systemic vasodilation improves the systemic blood flow and decreases the pulmonary flow, which may be advantageous in children with high pulmonary flows. Marked falls in systemic vascular resistance may cause the reversal of the shunt, with severe cyanosis and metabolic acidosis.

PERI-OPERATIVE MANAGEMENT

Pre-operative assessment

The aim of the pre-operative assessment is to determine the child's health, the adequacy of the medical management, and to decide upon the appropriate anaesthetic technique. In addition to the routine history and examination, particular attention should be paid to fluid balance, drug therapy (Chapter 5), ventricular failure, ventilatory failure, and blood gas analysis. Cardiac catheter and echocardiographic results provide information on ventricular pressures, function and size, the interconnection between the chambers, and the resistances of the systemic and pulmonary circulations. A coagulation screen may be abnormal, with polycythaemia and decreased platelet activity found in cyanotic heart disease, or with decreased clotting factor production caused by impaired liver function in right ventricular failure.

Anaesthetic management

Premedication for elective cardiac surgery should produce a sedated compliant child. The use of local anaesthetic cream has greatly facilitated intravenous induction of anaesthesia and should be part of the premedication schedule. Standard oral dosage regimens of chloral hydrate (20 mg kg^{-1}), triclofos (100 mg kg^{-1}), trimeprazine (2 mg kg^{-1}), diazepam (0.5 mg kg^{-1}) or midazolam (0.5 mg kg^{-1}) can be used. Midazolam can also be given rectally or intranasally. Dosages should be reduced or omitted in the very sick, those under one year of age, and if respiratory decompensation or obstruction is suspected.

Ideally a 22 G indwelling catheter is inserted painlessly into the sedated child prior to intravenous induction of anaesthesia. Induction is achieved using small doses of thiopentone (less than 2 mg kg^{-1}) if indicated, followed by fentanyl (10 μg kg^{-1}) repeated as required, and pancuronium (0.1 mg kg^{-1}). If intravenous access cannot be secured, gaseous induction with halothane or isoflurane and 50 per cent nitrous oxide in oxygen can be used.

Monitoring during induction consists of the maximum tolerated by the child. This usually comprises ECG, pulse oximeter, and precordial stethoscope, all of which provide valuable information. Nasal intubation with a plain PVC tube facilitates prolonged post-operative ventilation if required. A small air leak should be present during normal ventilation, and the endotracheal tube should be secured to allow easy suction of secretions through the tube and rapid changing in case of blockage. A nasogastric tube on free drainage will reduce the risk of aspiration of stomach contents past the uncuffed tube. Venous access is most easily provided by two 18 G or 20 G cannulae in the right internal jugular vein with a peripheral intravenous line for volume infusion. Large cannulae in small polycythaemic patients can predispose to thrombus formation. Intra-arterial blood pressure monitoring and arterial blood gas sampling are achieved by cannulation of either a radial or femoral artery.

Thermistors measuring oesophageal (blood) and nasopharyngeal (brain) temperature are required for cardiopulmonary by-pass management, but nasopharyngeal probes suffice for closed cardiac surgery. End tidal CO_2 monitoring is also valuable in the peri-operative period, and normocarbia is important in maintaining cerebral blood flow at the initiation of cardiopulmonary by-pass. The theoretical disadvantages of isoflurane in terms of small vessel vasodilation and 'coronary steal' are outweighed by the practical advantages of reduced myocardial depression, suppression of arrhythmias, and a reduction in cerebral metabolic rate for oxygen. Nitrous oxide should be used with caution in patients with right-to-left shunts to minimize systemic gaseous emboli. Serial arterial blood gas analysis should be made peri-operatively and FiO_2 and minute ventilation adjusted to produce adequate PaO_2. The tendency to acidosis that occurs during prolonged anaesthesia and surgery should be corrected using bolus injection of sodium bicarbonate based on blood gas analysis.

Cardiopulmonary by-pass

This technique is only employed for patients requiring open cardiac surgery. Palliative operations avoid the need for such intervention. After full heparinization (3 mg kg^{-1}), ventilation with 100 per cent oxygen, and arterial and venous cannulation, the patient may be placed on cardiopulmonary by-pass. Further doses of fentanyl and pancuronium can be given prior to this. Once the calculated full flow has been achieved, ventilation is unnecessary and is discontinued to facilitate surgery. The pump is primed with a mixture of fresh bank blood, human albumin solution, and Hartmann's solution to produce a haematocrit of between 25 and 30 per cent. At 37 °C full flow is 2.4 l m^{-2} min^{-1} but flow is reduced with temperature as oxygen consumption also falls with temperature. Venous cannulation is usually of the superior and inferior venae cavae with arterial cannulation at the aorta. More complex repairs, particularly re-operations, may require femoral venous to femoral arterial or left atrial to aortic cannulations.

Hypotension, occurring on by-pass (less than 40 mmHg) can be managed either by increasing flow or addition of a vasoconstrictor, such as metaraminol (0.5 mg) or phenylephrine (0.1 mg). Hypertension (greater than 70 mmHg) can be treated with fentanyl (1 μg kg^{-1}), glyceryltrinitrate (1 μg kg^{-1} min^{-1}), or sodium nitroprusside (0.3–1 μg kg^{-1} min^{-1}). For less complex cardiac surgery, cooling to 25–28 °C is sufficient to allow the operation to be safely completed. However, for more complex lesions, a period of low flow may be required for full evaluation and correction of the defect. This process takes advantage of the markedly reduced oxygen consumption of all organs occurring at these temperatures.

Total circulatory arrest can be carried out at temperatures below 20 °C, provided uniform body cooling has been established. This allows surgery to proceed on the most complex cardiac lesions, with the heart and great vessels drained of blood. The safe time limit of arrest is debated but less than 40 min is ideal. As all tissues are cold and no circulation is possible, re-warming does not occur and myocardial preservation is excellent. Cerebral protection can be maximized by placing ice packs around the head. Re-warming on cardiopulmonary by-pass usually requires the addition of sodium bicarbonate to correct metabolic acidosis and potassium chloride to correct hypokalaemia. Attention to these details prior to cessation of by-pass will reduce the likelihood of ventricular dysfunction and dysrhythmias imme-diately after cardiopulmonary by-pass. The temperature gradient should never exceed 15 °C anywhere in the by-pass circuit.

After removal of the aortic cross clamp and the commencement of cardiac action, the lungs are vigorously inflated to drive air from the lungs to the pulmonary veins and left atrium where it is aspirated. A temporary head-down position will reduce the risk of cerebral air embolus. The lungs are then ventilated normally.

Myocardial protection

This is achieved by cooling the myocardium prior to surgery, and in many centres an intra-aortic infusion of cardioplegic solution is employed. The fea-tures of this solution are that it should be cold (4 °C) and should stop the heart in asystole. This is achieved using a mixture of procainamide, potas-sium chloride, and magnesium chloride made up in Ringer's solution or added to colloid or blood. The cold cardioplegic solution (20 ml kg^{-1}) is infused under pressure (200–300 mmHg) into the aortic root after aortic cross clamping. At 30–40 min intervals, further doses of 10 ml kg^{-1} are repeated to maintain myocardial cooling and electrical silence. On removal of the aortic cross clamp, the cardioplegia is washed out of the coronary cir-culation and electrical activity rapidly returns.

MANAGEMENT OF SPECIFIC CONDITIONS

Patent ductus arteriosus (PDA)

A PDA produces a left-to-right shunt between the aorta and the pulmonary artery. The clinical presentation ranges from an incidental finding to that of left ventricular failure (LVF) caused by the increased pulmonary flow and excess volume load on the left ventricle. Ninety per cent of PDAs close within 9 weeks.

Peri-operative management is to assess the severity of heart failure and the need for supplemental oxygen or ventilation. Indomethacin (a prostaglandin synthetase inhibitor) may have been given to promote ductal closure. The anaesthetic technique requires full monitoring and is decided by the clinical condition of the child and the need for post-operative ventilation. Severely ill children show relative hypovolaemia, requiring caution with the use of inhalational agents and large doses of fentanyl. These children usually require ventilatory support after surgery. The surgical approach is through a left-thoracotomy, and during dissection vagal traction may cause bradycardia; recurrent laryngeal nerve damage can occur. Older children may have developed pulmonary hypertension which may increase blood loss from the pulmonary vasculature. Before ductal ligation, a trial clamping is performed when the murmur should disappear on oesophageal auscultation; during actual closure the blood pressure is electively decreased to reduce vessel wall tension.

Coarctation of the aorta

The narrowing of the aorta may be proximal, opposite, or distal to the origin of the ductus arteriosus. It produces proximal hypertension with left ventricular hypertrophy. The untreated condition is associated with an increased incidence of LVF, cerebrovascular accident, aortic dissection, and subacute bacterial endocarditis. The anatomical site of the coarctation determines the clinical presentation. In preductal stenosis, collateral vessels do not form during neonatal life, as blood flow to the lower body through the ductus arteriosus is adequate. Following closure of the ductus, the absence of collateral flow produces left ventricular pressure overload and early onset of heart failure. A persistent postductal stenosis requires the formation of collateral vessels during intra-uterine life to supply the lower body; following ductal closure there is adequate collateral flow and LVF rarely occurs.

Peri-operative management is to assess the severity and treatment of LVF. Prostaglandin E_1 may be used to minimize any LVF by maintaining the patency of the ductus until surgery. The presence of other congenital malformations should be sought. The anaesthetic management is a balance between minimizing LVF caused by pressure overload and the occurrence of lower body hypotension impairing spinal cord and renal perfusion. Full monitoring is required, including a *right* radial or brachial arterial catheter as the left subclavian artery may be intra-operatively clamped, as well as a femoral or pedal arterial catheter to monitor the lower body blood pressure.

Left ventricular function is affected by the closure of the ductus increasing the venous return to the left ventricle, and aortic cross clamping (required during the repair) increasing the afterload. Veno- and arteriolar dilators are manipulated to minimize the increases in filling pressures and systemic arterial blood pressure with constant attention to distal perfusion. Adequate perfusion of the spinal cord is dependent upon the collateral blood supply from the intercostal arteries and the radicular arteries. Distal pressures of greater than 50 mmHg reduce the risk of cord ischaemia. Repositioning of the aortic clamp to improve intercostal blood flow or a reduced dose of vasoactive drugs to increase the proximal driving pressure may improve distal pressures. The risk of neurological complication from spinal cord ischaemia is 0.5 per cent.[1]

Haemorrhage may occur during the repair and is exacerbated by the use of heparin (1 mg kg^{-1}) given to avoid thrombus formation during aortic cross clamping. Clamp release is associated with acute hypotension, the severity of which is decreased by accurate blood replacement, correction of acid–base imbalance, and the cessation of vasodilators prior to clamp release.

Post-operative persistent hypertension responds to appropriate anti-hypertensives (e.g. labetalol). Extubation after completion of surgery is preferred unless left ventricular and respiratory failure are present.

Vascular ring abnormalities

The abnormal development of the aortic arch and major vessels produces compression of the oesophagus and trachea, usually above the carina. The commonest malformation is a double aortic arch with either a small anterior or posterior limb.[2] An affected child presents with breathing difficulties exacerbated by feeding. The extent and site of the obstruction is assessed by clinical and radiological examination, and impaired pulmonary function may occur due to airway compression.

A gaseous induction is advisable because of the airway obstruction, the endotracheal tube being inserted beyond the obstruction. Haemorrhage can be severe, particularly with a posterior limb resection. Post-operative extubation is usual; if tracheomalacia is present, bronchoscopic assessment is required.

PALLIATIVE PROCEDURES

Systemic to pulmonary anastomosis

These procedures increase pulmonary blood flow and improve oxygenation by the creation of a systemic anastomosis with a pulmonary artery. The shunt palliates the reduced pulmonary blood flow of conditions such as pulmonary stenosis or atresia or tricuspid atresia. Full monitoring is required, with arterial and venous access sited on the contralateral side to the thoracotomy. Intra-operative problems are hypoxia and acidosis from compression of the lung, pulmonary artery clamping, and haemorrhage. The increased pulmonary blood flow can reduce pulmonary compliance and cause pulmonary oedema necessitating post-operative ventilation.

The commonest shunt performed is the Blalock–Taussig shunt, which is an anastomosis of the ipsilateral subclavian and pulmonary artery. The classical shunt sacrifices the subclavian artery, the modified shunt conserves the artery by using a synthetic graft.

The Waterston shunt, which is the anastomosis of the ascending aorta to the right pulmonary artery, may be used, but it is associated with deformation of the pulmonary artery, excessive pulmonary blood flow, and the occurrence of pulmonary hypertension.

Atrial septostomy

This procedure is used to create full systemic-venous mixing at the atrial level in palliation of transposition of the great vessels. The Rashkind procedure creates a large atrial septal defect by pulling the inflated balloon of a paediatric cardiac catheter back through the foramen ovale, thus disrupting the atrial septum. It is usually performed under general anaesthesia with full monitoring. However, advances with echocardiographic control of catheter placement may allow the septostomy to be performed under sedation.

OPEN CARDIAC SURGERY

Atrial septal defect (ASD)

An ASD is usually associated with a left-to-right shunt and may have few clinical manifestations. Repair of symptomatic ASDs or those with abnormal cardiac catheter data are easily undertaken and have few complications. The commonest of these is supraventricular dysrhythmias, including atrial fibrillation, atrial flutter, and nodal rhythms.

Ventricular septal defect (VSD)

Abnormal communications between the right and left ventricles can be so small that they will close spontaneously, but they may be large enough to present with high output cardiac failure in early life. A significant VSD should be closed prior to the development of pulmonary hypertension or heart failure, usually before 1 year of age. Repair undertaken through the tricuspid valve avoids right ventriculotomy with associated post-operative right ventricular dysfunction. Other complications include residual VSD and conducting tissue damage with dysrhythmias.

Atrioventricular canal defect

Complete atrioventricular canal defects are always associated with abnormalities of the tricuspid and mitral valves with both an interatrial and interven-

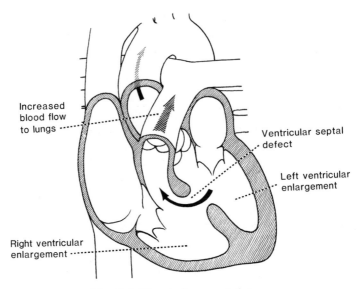

Fig. 7.2 Ventricular septal defect.

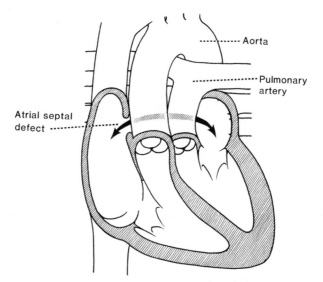

Fig. 7.3 Transposition with palliative atrial septal defect.

tricular communication.[3] Consequently, the four heart chambers are in communication and pulmonary hypertension can occur. Surgery must repair both the mitral and tricuspid valves, as well as patching the interatrial and interventricular defects. Surgery for partial atrioventricular canal defects must be directed to the interatrial communication and the mitral valve. Post-operative complications of both conditions include damage to the conducting tissue with supraventricular tachycardias and nodal rhythms, as well as atrioventricular valve regurgitation and heart failure requiring mechanical ventilation and inotropic drugs.

Transposition of the great arteries (TGA)

This condition is a result of malposition of the aorta and pulmonary arteries and requires a communication between the pulmonary and systemic circulations for postnatal survival.[4] If such a communication is small (usually a VSD), profound hypoxia, acidosis, and hypoglycaemia will be present and a Rashkind's atrial septostomy may improve oxygenation prior to definitive surgery. Larger communications between the circulations, while improving systemic oxygenation, may lead to heart failure and pulmonary oedema.

Operative interventions can either be directed to the arterial or venous (atrial) sides of the circulation. An arterial 'switch' operation performed early in life is curative and requires the anatomical re-siting of the aorta on to the systemic ventricle, with accompanying coronary arteries and the pulmonary artery on to the pulmonary ventricle. A successful operation requires minimal post-operative inotropic support. The complications of bleeding, coronary artery obstruction with myocardial ischaemia and infarction can disrupt the peri-operative period. Atrial redirection is achieved by either a Senning or a Mustard operation when systemic venous blood is directed into the systemic ventricle and the pulmonary venous blood is directed into the pulmonary ventricle. Complications with these operations are related to bleeding, obstruction of the venous pathways, rhythm disturbances, and decreased right (systemic) ventricular function post-operatively.

Anomalous pulmonary venous drainage (TAPVD)

The term covers both partial and total anomalous pulmonary venous drainage. The former can be of minor severity, requiring correction of the atrial septum at operation. The latter requires mixing of the systemic and pulmonary circulation at atrial level for survival. Four types are described according to the anatomical site of entry of the pulmonary veins into the systemic venous circulation.[5] Supracardiac TAPVD is most common, with drainage to the left innominate vein or the superior vena cava. Intracardiac TAPVD may be via the right atrium or coronary sinus, and infracardiac TAPVD can be via the portal or hepatic veins, ductus venosus, or inferior vena cava. This latter condition may be subdivided into supra- or infra-diaphragmatic types. The fourth classification covers anomalous PVD at two or more sites. Pulmonary venous obstruction is commonly seen with the anatomical defect and leads to pulmonary hypertension, pulmonary oedema, severe hypoxia, cyanosis, acidosis, and hypoglycaemia. Severity of illness pre-operatively is reflected in a high peri-operative mortality (*c*. 30 per cent) with a requirement for mechanical ventilation and high dose inotropes post-operatively.

Tetralogy of Fallot

The four original anatomical features described were a ventricular septal defect, pulmonary valvular stenosis, overriding aorta, and right ventricular hypertrophy. These have been modified to include right ventricular outflow tract (RVOT) obstruction involving at least one of the following, the infundibulum, the pulmonary valve, or valve ring, and the pulmonary artery.

Patients with this condition may exhibit pulmonary artery spasm when the RVOT undergoes constriction; the so-called cyanotic spell. This causes increased right-to-left shunting through the VSD and systemic desaturation and hypoxia. Patients with cyanotic spells receive oral popranolol to dilate the RVOT and should continue therapy until operation. Stimuli to RVOT constriction include light anaesthesia and handling of the heart. Immediate management includes increasing the depth of anaesthesia with halothane, an intravenous fluid load (1–2 ml kg^{-1}), and an intravenous bolus of sodium bicarbonate (1 mmol kg^{-1}). If RVOT constriction persists, propranolol (up to 0.1 mg kg^{-1}) will dilate the RVOT and restore systemic saturation. The systemic arterial blood pressure is well maintained throughout and after treatment of cyanotic episodes. Palliation for tetralogy of Fallot is by a systemic to

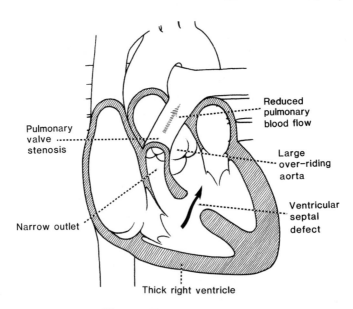

Fig. 7.4 Tetralogy of Fallot.

pulmonary shunt, but complete repair in infancy is optimal if the anatomy is favourable. Intractable spasm at operation requires rapid cannulation and commencement of cardiopulmonary by-pass.

Pulmonary hypertension

Left-to-right shunt in the infant if associated with a high pulmonary blood flow can predispose to pulmonary hypertension. This is characterized by a pulmonary artery (PA) pressure above 50 per cent of systemic at the end of cardiopulmonary by-pass. Pulmonary vascular crisis after by-pass occurs when the PA pressure rises to systemic level with a subsequent fall in arterial oxygen saturation and later systemic arterial pressure. Prophylactic treatment of at-risk patients is with phenoxybenzamine ($0.5-1$ mg kg^{-1}) before cardiopulmonary by-pass and intravenously 8 hourly afterwards, and is best used in conjunction with full mechanical ventilation to a PCO_2 of 30 mmHg and PaO_2 greater than 100 mmHg. Sedation with a fentanyl infusion (0.1 μg kg^{-1} min^{-1}) will obtund the pulmonary vascular response to airway toilet and handling, although these should be minimized during this period. Crises occurring on phenoxybenzamine treatment require the addition of prostacyclin ($5-20$ mg kg^{-1} min^{-1}) by intravenous infusion.

POST-OPERATIVE MANAGEMENT

After the completion of surgery and re-warming on cardiopulmonary by-pass, the patient is weaned from the by-pass machine. Ideally, a right atrial pressure of $8-12$ mmHg with a left atrial pressure of less than 10 mmHg will be accompanied by a systemic arterial pressure of $70-80$ mmHg. Some patients may manifest signs of heart failure, with a rising central venous pressure or left atrial pressure and falling systemic arterial pressure. These patients will require the addition of inotropic infusions.

Inotropic drugs

The most commonly used inotrope is dopamine, with doses up to 5 μg kg^{-1} min^{-1} producing diuresis and natriuresis and doses of $5-10$ μg kg^{-1} min^{-1} adding inotropic action. Dobutamine in similar or higher doses represents a rational choice for patients after cardiac surgery, combining an inotropic action with systemic vasodilation. Adrenaline may be required in doses from $0.01-0.5$ μg kg^{-1} min^{-1}. The peripheral vasoconstriction produced by an adrenaline infusion is usually offset by an infusion of glyceryl trinitrate ($0.5-5$ μg kg^{-1} min^{-1}).

Phosphodiesterase inhibitors

The phosphodiesterase (PDE) inhibitors enoximone and milrinone have a synergistic effect with β_1 agonists. Both groups of drugs act to raise intracellular cyclic AMP in muscle cells. The PDE inhibitors also exert a peripheral vasodilatatory action and are ideal in combination with adrenaline in severe heart failure. (An initial dose of 0.5 mg kg^{-1} of enoximone at the time of removal of the aortic cross-clamp followed by an infusion of 2–5 μg kg^{-1} min^{-1} reduces the requirement for other inotropes and increases cardiac index in adults.)[6]

When haemodynamic stability has been achieved, protamine can be given to reverse the effect of the heparin, and doses of 3 mg kg^{-1} are usually sufficient. A rapid infusion of blood may be required during the administration of protamine, as the drug is a systemic vasodilator, although a pulmonary vasoconstrictor. Blood products aiding haemostasis which may be used at this stage include fresh frozen plasma, cryoprecipitate, and platelet transfusion. Post-operatively the patients are transferred with their infusions and full monitoring in place to the intensive care unit. Here they may be weaned from their inotropic support and mechanical ventilation prior to extubation.

REFERENCES

1. Brewer, L. A. III *et al.* (1972). Spinal cord complications following surgery for coarctation of the aorta; a study of 66 cases. *Journal of Thoracic and Cardiovascular Surgery*, **64**, 368.
2. Hendren, W. H. and Kim, S. H. (1978). Paediatric thoracic surgery. In *Pulmonary disease of the fetus, newborn and child* (ed. E. M. Scarpelli, A. P. M. Auld, and H. S. Goldman), p. 166. Lea & Febiger, Philadelphia.
3. Rastelli, G. C., Kirklin, J. W., and Titus, J. L. (1976). Anatomic observations on complete forms of persistent common atrioventricular canal with special reference to atrioventricular valves. *Mayo Clinic Proceedings*, **41**, 296.
4. Beynen, F. M. and Tarhan, S. (1989). Anaesthesia for the surgical repair of congenital heart defects in children. In *Cardiovascular anaesthesia and postoperative care* (2nd edn) (ed. S. Tarhan), p. 183. Year Book Medical, London.
5. Lucas, R. V. Jr and Schmidt, R. E. (1977). Anomolous venous connections, pulmonary and systemic. In *Heart disease in infants, children and adolescents* (2nd edn) (ed. A. J. Moss, F. H. Adams, and G. C. Emmanouilides), p. 437. Williams & Wilkins, Baltimore.
6. Boldt, J., Knothe, C., Zickmann, B. *et al.* (1992). The role of enoximone in cardiac surgery. *British Journal of Anaesthesia*, **69**, 45.

FURTHER READING

Beynen, F.A. and Tarhan, S. (1989). Anaesthesia for the surgical repair of congenital heart defects in children. In *Cardiovascular anaesthesia and postoperative care* (2nd edn) (ed. S. Tarhan), pp. 105–212. Year Book Medical, London.

Sumner, E. (1989). Anaesthesia for patients with cardiac disease. In *Textbook of paediatric anaesthetic practice* (ed. E. Sumner and D. J. Hatch), pp. 305–38. Baillière Tindall, London.

Eyres, R. (1995). The management of neonatal cardiac conditions. In *A handbook of neonatal anaesthesia* (ed. D. G. Hughes, S. J. Mather and A. R. Wolf) Chapter 12. W. B. Saunders, London.

8

Anaesthesia for specialist surgery

D. G. Hughes

GENERAL AND UROLOGICAL SURGERY

Many children undergo elective surgery, ranging in age from the preterm to the fullterm neonate, infant, child, and adolescent. Occasionally the underlying pathology results in the child being admitted as an emergency. In the congenital conditions seen in the neonatal period most of the surgery is carried out on a semi-urgent basis. This chapter has been divided into three sections: elective surgical conditions, emergency surgical conditions, and congenital defects found in the neonatal period.

ELECTIVE GENERAL CONDITIONS

Tumour surgery

Wilms' tumour (nephroblastoma)
Neuroblastoma
Liver tumours
Phaeochromocytoma } very rare
Teratoma

Some of these tumours may require emergency anaesthesia for investigations, e.g. bone marrow and radiological investigation. Insertion of a 'long' (central venous) line is commonly carried out for intravenous feeding and for drug therapy in these children.

Removal of thyroglossal cyst or branchial cyst

There are a number of lesions in the head and neck region only found in children. The main problem is access and these children require intubation. Local infiltration of bupivacaine provides excellent post-operative analgesia.

Elective urological surgery

Diagnostic
Cystocopy, ureteric catheterization.

Surgical
> Kidneys: congenital abnormalities of the kidney and urinary tract may require surgical correction, e.g. nephrectomy, pyeloplasty.
> Urinary tract: reimplantation of ureters.
> Hypospadias surgery: the urethra does not reach the glans penis and opens on the ventral surface of the penis.
> Orchiopexy.
> Circumcision.

Most of the children undergoing elective urological procedures have good renal function, and similar anaesthetic techniques can be used for general surgery and urological surgery. Many procedures can be carried out on an out-patient basis and should be encouraged. Most of the procedures are best carried out using a combination of general anaesthesia and appropriate regional analgesic techniques, e.g. penile block, caudal or lumbar epidural block (see Chapter 11). The operations are usually of short duration, the common procedures being inguinal herniotomy, orchidopexy, circumcision, and minor hypospadias surgery. All these procedures can be carried out as day cases.

The major urological procedures are straightforward although careful positioning of the child is important. Blood loss may be significant. Postoperatively great care must be taken with all the catheters and drains that urological surgeons usually require. Pain in these children can be very well controlled using regional analgesic techniques, caudal or lumbar epidurals, with continuous infusion of local anaesthetic agents (see p. 227).

The management of children who have poor renal function or are in renal failure is discussed in Chapter 6. Obviously these children could present for any surgical operation and not just for urological surgery.

Specific surgical conditions

Wilms' tumour (nephroblastoma)

This is one of the most common malignant tumours occurring in childhood, usually presenting before the age of 5 years, commonly as a large abdominal mass which is bilateral in 5 per cent of cases and is often associated with other renal abnormalities. The child may be hypertensive, either due to compression of the renal artery or due to the secretion of renin, and is often anaemic. As already discussed they may require urgent investigations, e.g. bone barrow, biopsy, insertion of long line, and renal angiograms (to check on possible extension of the tumour into the inferior vena cava).

The main problems encountered are:

- very large tumours may splint the diaphragm;
- the inferior vena cava (IVC) may be obstructed by manipulation of the tumour during surgery;
- large blood loss;
- blood pressure changes.

The intravenous infusion must be in the upper part of the body because of possible IVC obstruction, and a central line should be inserted into an internal jugular or subclavian vein. Close observation of the blood pressure is needed while the tumour is being manipulated since IVC obstruction may occur.

Neuroblastoma

This is a retroperitoneal tumour arising from the sympathetic nervous system, adrenal medulla, or paravertebral ganglia. It is a very malignant tumour which again usually presents before the age of 5 years, and can involve the spinal cord by compression and metastasises to the liver, brain, and bone marrow. Most (90 per cent) of these children have a raised vanillyl mandelic acid (VMA) level but only a few tumours secrete adrenalin and noradrenalin and it is only these children who may show signs of excessive catecholamine secretion: hypertension, tachycardia, and pallor. The problems encountered are very similar to those occurring in Wilms' tumours, i.e. a large abdominal mass resulting in similar surgical problems although with no danger of IVC embolization.

Phaeochromocytoma

A very rare tumour in children which presents with symptoms associated with excess secretion of the catecholamines adrenalin and noradrenalin, i.e. headache, nausea, and vomiting, and persistent hypertension which may occasionally be paroxysmal. The anaesthetic is especially dangerous if the child is not properly prepared pre-operatively. Vasoconstriction which occurs as a result of the excess secretion of noradrenalin results in a contracted intravascular volume. The child may be pretreated with an alpha blocker, e.g. phenoxybenzamine but since administration of phenoxybenzamine actually results in destruction of α-receptors this should be stopped 2 weeks prior to surgery and control of blood pressure established with another agent. Regrowth of α-receptors allows response to α-agonist drugs to maintain blood pressure after the tumour has been removed.

Tachycardia and tachyarrhythmias are due to the overproduction of adrenalin. It may be necessary to use beta-blockade to control these arrhythmias. Good premedication is essential to reduce anxiety, and all drugs that result in catecholamine release must be avoided during surgery. Suxamethonium may increase the release of catecholamines, and halothane should be avoided because of its arrhythmogenic effect. Any drug that releases histamine, e.g. tubocurarine, should not be used. Vecuronium and fentanyl infusion would seem the ideal choice, together with enflurane or isoflurane. Handling of the tumour intra-operatively may cause a rise in blood pressure which can be controlled with sodium nitroprusside. Lignocaine can be used to treat ventricular arrhythmias if they occur.

ACUTE EMERGENCY PROCEDURES

Acute appendicitis
Perforated Meckel's diverticulum
Intussusception
Torsion of the testicle

None of these emergency procedures should be carried out until appropriate correction of electrolytes and rehydration has taken place, i.e. check electrolytes, urine output, and fluid replacement. If the obstruction is above the duodenum, vomiting will lead to a loss of hydrogen ions, chloride, potassium, and sodium. If below the duodenum, the vomiting will be bile-stained but the acid-base upset will not be as marked. Diarrhoea is also a major cause of fluid and electrolyte loss in children, especially potassium. The child may also be dehydrated due to large intraperitoneal losses of fluid which will cause abdominal distension and may lead to diaphragmatic splinting in small infants. Circulating volume depletion should be replaced by colloid (4.5 per cent human albumen), together with appropriate crystalloid infusion to replace sodium and potassium loss. A nasogastric tube should be passed and left on free drainage, nasogastric losses being replaced intravenously as 0.9 per cent sodium chloride.

The anaesthetic management is the same as for any emergency procedure, i.e. avoidance of gastric regurgitation and subsequent aspiration. Even though there is a nasogastric tube *in situ* the child has an ileus and may well still have a full stomach. It is essential to check that the intravenous infusion is reliable since they are often well hidden under bandages. Pre-oxygenation of 3–4 min is always attempted using a close-fitting mask. If the child is frightened, a cupped hand can be used but full denitrogenation cannot then be achieved. This is followed by a rapid induction/intubation sequence with cricoid pressure using thiopentone or propofol, atropine if indicated, and suxamethonium. Once the endotracheal tube is in place, the anaesthetic can be continued with oxygen and air, muscle relaxant, and appropriate analgesic drugs and volatile agents. Nitrous oxide should be avoided in bowel surgery. Abdominal closure is always assisted by decompression of the bowel and this lessens the dangers of post-operative diaphragmatic splinting. The child should be extubated on his side once the airway reflexes have returned.

Intussusception

Intussusception is the most frequent cause of obstruction in the first year of life. In this condition one piece of bowel is invaginated into another and often the infant appears to be deceptively well. In the early stages it is possible to reduce the obstruction with a barium enema in 75 per cent of cases. Hydrostatic reduction with barium is being superseded by pneumatic reduction (air enema) which has a 90 per cent success rate. If this fails it is essential to perform a laparotomy because the bowel may become damaged and resection of part of the intestine may be necessary.

Often in intussusception large volumes of fluid are lost into the bowel and up to 40 ml kg^{-1} of colloid may be needed to restore the circulating volume prior to surgery.

Torsion of the testicle

This is one of the few conditions that requires urgent surgery. Again the child has to be treated as an emergency case with the possibility of a full stomach, i.e. rapid sequence induction, and not an inhalational technique using a mask.

Torsion occasionally occurs in neonates but is more common in older children. Operation to fix the testis is relatively urgent to avoid necrosis. The second testis should also be fixed. Such surgery presents no particular anaesthetic problems but relief of considerable pre-operative pain may be required. Torsion of the body of the testis may be confused with torsion of the hydatid of Morgagni, which occurs frequently.

SURGICAL CONDITIONS ENCOUNTERED IN THE NEONATE AND SMALL INFANT

In Britain, major surgery on neonates and small infants is largely restricted to the regional centres with specialist facilities. Some common conditions, for example congenital pyloric stenosis and herniotomy, can be safely managed in district hospitals provided staff are trained and experienced in the techniques, and that there are facilities for post-operative paediatric nursing care. Other, more serious problems require the facilities of a major regional centre for intensive nursing and medical care.

Congenital hypertrophic pyloric stenosis

This condition is common, occurring in about one in 400 live births. The majority of affected infants are male. The pathological process is thickening of the muscle of the pylorus, causing obstruction to the passage of food from the stomach into the duodenum. The infant begins to vomit regularly in the first few weeks of life, the vomiting becoming projectile. Weight loss, dehydration, and alkalosis with hypochloraemia is inevitable without treatment. Usually gastric peristalsis is visible following a feed and a *tumour* or lump can be felt in most cases.

This condition is not a surgical emergency and the infant must be rehydrated and normal electrolyte balance restored before surgery is undertaken. Usually sodium, chloride, and potassium replacement is required. The alkalosis may not be fully corrected unless the chloride value is as high as 105 mM l^{-1}. Operation should be referred if it is less than 95 mM l^{-1}.

The stomach should be washed out regularly and drained through a gastric tube. Premedication is not required, although atropine is sometimes prescribed to reduce salivary secretions. The gastric tube should be aspirated immediately prior to induction of anaesthesia, which may be performed through the intravenous infusion established earlier for rehydration. The nasogastric tube should be left open during the induction. A rapid sequence induction technique should be performed with cricoid pressure. Anaesthesia can be maintained using air, oxygen, muscle relaxant and a volatile agent.

The operation consists of splitting the muscle of the pylorus down to the mucosa (Ramstedt's procedure). Feeding is re-established quickly after operation and the procedure itself results in very little physiological disturbance. Post-operative analgesia is provided by wound infiltration with a local anaesthetic and rectal or nasogastric paracetamol.

Inguinal herniotomy

Inguinal hernia is commonly due to a patent processus vaginalis. Premature babies have a high incidence of inguinal hernia. The hernia is usually reducible and patients rarely present with dehydration due to intestinal obstruction. Surgery is carried out as an elective procedure. If however, obstruction has occurred, meticulous attention must be given to rehydration and pre-operative preparation. Operation will be planned urgently if the bowel is at risk from ischaemia. Such patients are at risk from regurgitation and aspiration pneumonitis. Pre-oxygenation and cricoid pressure should be employed. The majority of cases, however, are healthy and may be managed as elective procedures with inhalational anaesthesia or with controlled ventilation using a muscle relaxant.

Small infants (less than 1 year of age) should be intubated because traction on the peritoneum may provoke both laryngeal spasm and reflex bradycardias. Light anaesthesia must be avoided. Blockade of the ilio-inguinal nerve or caudal epidural block provides good post-operative pain relief. Ilioinguinal and iliohypogastric nerve block ('iliac crest block') provides only cutaneous analgesia and will not prevent vagal reflexes due to traction on peritoneal structures. To be effective, caudal epidural block to T10 is required with a volume of local anaesthetic of not less than 1.25 ml kg^{-1}. This may produce significant weakness of the legs.

Intestinal obstruction

In neonates, intestinal obstruction is a common surgical emergency occurring in one per 1500 births. The commonest causes are duodenal atresia, jejunal and ileal atresias, volvulus, meconium ileus (seen in about 10 per cent of cystic fibrosis patients), and Hirschsprung's disease. These children often present with vomiting, abdominal distension occasionally interfering with respiration, and failure to pass faeces. Meticulous attention to fluid replacement is essential in all cases of intestinal obstruction, correcting electrolyte imbalance and restoring circulating volume with colloid.

Anaesthesia for these conditions is similar and precautions for a full stomach including aspiration of the nasogastric tube prior to induction and pre-oxygenation (prior to applying cricoid pressure) should be employed. A muscle relaxant technique is used. During surgery any handling of the gut may cause further periods of hypotension requiring large volumes of colloid (plasma or blood). Decompression of the bowel can result in the contents being regurgitated into the mouth, even with a nasogastric tube in place. Great care must be taken during this procedure to aspirate the gastric tube. A large bore tube should be used during surgery, e.g. 12 F.G., which can be replaced by a normal nasogastric tube at the end of surgery.

Exomphalos and gastroschisis

Exomphalos (omphalocele) is a condition where the abdominal contents herniate into the umbilical cord. The covering membrane may rupture before or after birth. The incidence is about one in 5000 live births. Gastroschisis is a defect of the abdominal wall itself, lateral to the umbilicus, and occurs more frequently on the right side. It is less common than exomphalos, with an incidence of one in 30 000 live births. Both conditions may be associated with other gut abnormalities, genito-urinary malformations, and cardiac defects. In both conditions it is necessary to replace the contents into the abdomen as soon as possible. The procedure is probably one of the very few absolute neonatal emergencies, i.e. should be operated on within 5–6 hours of birth. There is an associated large protein loss and any delay may result in infection. Occasionally, replacing all the contents of the sac in the abdomen impairs respiration and the infant will require a short period of post-operative ventilation. Sometimes it is not possible to replace all the contents in the abdomen. They are then placed in a silastic pouch stitched to the abdominal wall and can be gradually pushed back into the abdomen, over a short period of time. This technique does not impair ventilation and the infant can breathe spontaneously post-operatively. However there is often a prolonged ileus and all these infants require parenteral nutrition through a 'long' line inserted at the end of the operation. The legs should be avoided for infusions because there is impaired venous return and a danger of oedema of the lower body.

Imperforate anus

Anal or rectal anomalies occur in about one in 5000 live births. There are many different degrees of abnormality, some of which may need a simple anoplasty, whereas a more complex procedure such as colostomy may be required if anal agnesis is present. The anaesthetic management of these conditions is uncomplicated and good intra- and post-operative analgesia can be achieved with 'single shot' caudal epidurals using local anaesthetic combined with an opioid.

Congenital diaphragmatic hernia

This condition is fairly rare, occurring in only one in 4000 live births and presents shortly after birth. The hernia is more common on the left side and is associated with hypoplasia of the lung on that side. There may be profound respiratory distress with increasing tachypnoea, cyanosis, and acidosis. The child often displays a flattened abdomen because some of the gut is in the chest cavity. Other associated problems such as malrotation of the gut and congenital heart disease may also occur. The diagnosis can be confirmed by a chest/abdomen X-ray. Once the diagnosis is established, further management depends on the degree of respiratory embarrassment. Even with modern treatment overall mortality may approach 50 per cent. A nasogastric tube should be passed to deflate the stomach. Severe respiratory distress will require intermittent positive pressure ventilation (IPPV). However, positive pressure face-mask ventilation should be avoided since this will cause further distension of the stomach. Inflation pressures should be kept as low as possible to avoid the danger of pneumothorax.

Previously it was thought that these children should be operated on immediately, to relieve the compression on the lung.[1] However, it is now realized that the infant should be stabilized for up to 24 hours prior to surgery using IPPV with muscle relaxants and a morphine infusion. A preductal arterial line in the right arm and a postductal arterial line (umbilical) should ideally be used to determine the degree of ductal shunting due to pulmonary hypertension (persistent fetal circulation), remembering also that shunting can take place at atrial level. Tolazoline and prostacyclin by infusion have been used to treat pulmonary hypertension. Colloid and occasionally a dopamine or dobutamine infusion may be required to maintain systemic blood pressure. A laparotomy is carried out, when the infant is as stable as possible, to remove the intestinal contents from the thorax and to close the defect in the diaphragm. Although most of the herniae are left-sided, through the foramen of Bochdalek, herniation can occur on either side. Sometimes there is agenesis of the diaphragm and the large defect needs to be patched with a synthetic mesh. The repaired diaphragm cannot contract and there may then be paradoxical movement of that portion of the diaphragm during spontaneous ventilation. The post-operative management of these infants is complex and requires close observation and monitoring for many days or weeks. Prolonged artificial ventilation may be required and currently IPPV together with negative pressure tanks (CNEP) and high frequency oscillation are all used in the weaning of these infants from respiratory support. Extracorporeal membrane oxygenation (ECMO) has been tried but probably provides little extra benefit and has a high incidence of complications, e.g. severe bleeding. Research is currently in progress into the use of inhaled nitric oxide in this condition. Overall mortality is about 50 per cent and has changed little in recent years.

Oesophageal atresia and tracheo-oesophageal fistula

The incidence of oesophageal atresia is about one in 3000 live births. In the vast majority of cases there is a distal fistula between the trachea and the oesophagus with a blind-ending upper oesophageal pouch (type IIIb, see Fig. 8.1). There may also be heart, renal and gut anomalies. The condition is associated with polyhydramnios and the onset of premature labour. The infant may be unable to swallow any saliva, which drools from the mouth. There is an obvious risk of aspiration of this saliva into the lungs, with subsequent pneumonia. The diagnosis of atresia is confirmed if a catheter cannot be passed into the stomach.

The main problems in this condition arise from aspiration of stomach contents into the tracheobronchial tree through the fistula, or from spill-over of secretions from a blind-ending upper oesophageal pouch. Initial management consists of draining the pouch through a double-lumen Replogle tube, physiotherapy, and, if necessary, antibiotics. The infant should be nursed prone. The diagnosis should never be confirmed by using barium studies because this may result in further pulmonary aspiration.

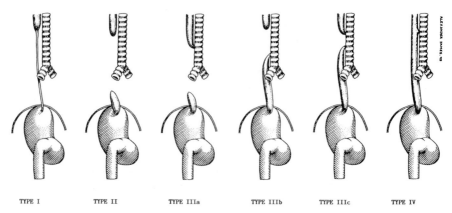

| TYPE I | TYPE II | TYPE IIIa | TYPE IIIb | TYPE IIIc | TYPE IV |

Fig. 8.1 Types of tracheo-oesophageal fistula (after an original drawing by J. E. Hughes)

A plain X-ray will show the catheter in the upper pouch with the presence of air in the stomach.

It has been suggested that intubation should be carried out with the baby breathing spontaneously. However, most anaesthetists intubate using muscle relaxants together with gentle ventilation throughout the operation. Careful positioning of the endotracheal tube is important because the fistula is situated on the posterior tracheal wall 1 or 2 cm above the carina. Excessive inflation pressures must be avoided. The fistula is tied off first using an extrapleural approach through the right thorax. The upper pouch is surgically identified by pushing a nasogastric tube down into the pouch. Once the fistula is tied off, the anaesthetic becomes easier because the problems of distending the stomach with anaesthetic gases passing through the fistula are resolved. If possible, primary oesophageal repair is carried out and a nasogastric tube is passed through the anastomosis into the stomach. Some surgeons create a gastrotomy and pass a transpyloric feeding tube. Most of these infants do not need to be ventilated post-operatively.

Neonatal necrotizing enterocolitis (NEC)

NEC is not a congenital disease but is seen particularly in premature infants. It results from ischaemia of the wall of the intestine and can result in perforation and peritonitis. The cause is unknown but it is thought to be associated with asphyxia at birth, catheterization of the umbilical artery, major stress, and exchange transfusions. Infants present with simple gastro-intestinal disturbances which may lead to peritonitis with a distended abdomen, ileus, and bloody stools. An abdominal X-ray shows gas in the wall of the bowel (pneumatosis intestinalis). Usually these children are managed medically but may need surgery. The anaesthetic problems are not only related to NEC but also to conditions associated with the premature neonate, respiratory distress syndrome, and apnoea. Blood and fluid volumes need to be restored and acid–base balance needs to be corrected, perhaps with pre-operative ventilation. In these premature neonates it is essential to avoid nitrous oxide because it may increase the size of the intramural gas in the bowel. However, high concentrations of inspired oxygen should also be avoided and an air, oxygen, fentanyl, muscle relaxant technique should ideally be used, the inspired oxygen concentration being titrated to achieve an oxygen saturation of 95%. Opioid analgesics can be used because these infants will be ventilated post-operatively.

EAR, NOSE, AND THROAT SURGERY (ENT) — OTORHINOLARYNGOLOGY

Many ENT procedures are carried out on children in ENT or district general hospitals and not in children's hospitals and it is essential that a children's ward is available. Many operations can result in blood in the nasopharynx post-operatively. The airway is often shared by the surgeon and meticulous attention must be taken to avoid kinking, disconnections, or even extubation. The post-operative management of these children requires skilled nursing care both in the recovery room and on the ward.

Diagnostic procedures in small babies such as microlaryngoscopy require considerable skill on the part of the operating team, and new developments for the treatment of lesions of the larynx using laser technology has resulted in additional anaesthetic problems.

Adenotonsillectomy

This is one of the commonest operations carried out on children, either adenoidectomy with myringotomies or the combination with tonsillectomy.

Usually a volatile agent technique with either spontaneous or controlled ventilation is used, supplemented by low-dose opioid and non-steroidal analgesics.

Obstructive sleep apnoea

Patients presenting with this condition are usually young children and are referred because of snoring, somnolence, and airway obstruction. The diagnosis is usually made by the time the anaesthetist first sees the patient, unless he/she is involved with polygraphic sleep studies (usually haemoglobin saturation and thoracic impedence pneumography). The tonsils may not be particularly large.

Presentation

- commonest age 2–6 years
- snoring or partial airway obstruction when awake
- tend to be obese
- daytime somnolence
- nocturnal apnoea
- failure to thrive
- chest infections
- craniofacial anomalies
- neurological problems

Pathology

The anatomical abnormalities lead to a partially obstructed upper airway, worsened by obesity, a large tongue, and a supine sleeping position. Brain stem neurological dysfunction with abnormal control of pharyngeal and laryngeal musculature leads to partial collapse of the airway on inspiration.

Hypoxia and hypercarbia eventually lead to pulmonary hypertension and severe cases can develop right heart failure (cor pulmonale), with right ventricular hypertrophy.

Diagnosis

- history
- ENT examination (including nasendoscopy)
- polygraphic sleep studies showing periods of apnoea and desaturation

Treatment
Adenotonsillectomy.

Pre-operative assessment
Particular attention should be paid to associated medical conditions, a history of recent upper respiratory or chest infection, and current medication.

Physical examination must assess respiratory function and the possibility of a difficult airway at induction or intubation.

Pre-operative inspection of the tonsils and pharynx is useful. Careful cardiovascular examination is required.

Investigations
No particular investigations over and above those for any tonsillectomy (haemoglobin concentration) are required unless there is clinical evidence of a chest infection (chest radiograph) or heart failure (chest radiograph or ECG).

Pre-operative preparation
Good rapport is essential to gain the child's confidence. A visit to the hospital to familiarize the child with the ward helps to allay anxiety.

SEDATIVE PREMEDICATION SHOULD BE AVOIDED

Anaesthetic management
- As for routine tonsillectomy except that inhalational induction is preferred using high concentrations of oxygen.
- The glottis should be visualized before a muscle relaxant is given.
- These patients should remain in the recovery room or go to a high dependency area post-operatively until the effects of anaesthesia have worn off.

PREDISPOSING CONDITIONS IN OBSTRUCTIVE SLEEP APNOEA

Adenotonsillar hypertrophy

Micrognathia
     e.g.   Pierre Robin anomalad
                     Treacher Collins syndrome
                     Goldenhar's syndrome
                     Moebius' syndrome

Other craniofacial anomalies
     e.g.   Down's syndrome (trisomy 21)
                     Acromegaly
                     Prader–Willi syndrome

Neuromuscular disorders
     e.g.   Arnold–Chiari malformation
                     Bulbar palsy
                     Cerebral palsy

Occasionally a child with grossly enlarged tonsils may present with severe airway obstruction and stridor and will require elective intubation and treatment prior to adenotonsillectomy. Opioids should be used with care.

Problems for the anaesthetist
- competition for the airway with the surgeon;
- the chronic conditions already discussed and their sequelae;
- may be bleeding post-operatively.

The anaesthetic technique used is straightforward, with gaseous or intravenous induction followed by intubation using suxamethonium, mivacurium or halothane and allowing the child to breathe spontaneously during the procedure. Sedative premedication should be avoided if there is severe airway obstruction or symptoms of obstructive sleep apnoea. Appropriate doses of analgesics such as *low dose* opioids or diclofenac[2] should be given. Many anaesthetists use a combination of both of these. Large doses of opioids are unnecessary and carry a risk of increased post-operative apnoea in children with sleep apnoea syndrome. They also greatly increase the incidence of post-operative vomiting. Only rarely is more than 50 μg kg^{-1} of morphine required when given in combination with a non-steroidal anti-inflammatory analgesic.

Post-tonsillectomy bleeding

Diagnosis of this condition is dependent on a high level of suspicion in the recovery ward and on the general ward. Post-operatively an indwelling intravenous cannula should be left in a vein. If necessary, blood can be taken early for grouping and 'save serum'.

The main problems include:

- swallowed blood with possible vomiting on induction;
- hypovolaemia shown by a tachycardia with cold extremities.

The child must be resuscitated with intravenous fluid pre-operatively; blood must be cross-matched and be available prior to surgery. Blood loss during tonsillectomy may be significant in a small child. Such children should receive intravenous fluid electively during tonsillectomy (0.9% saline or Hartmann's solution, not glucose).

Anaesthetic management

The technique used depends on the age of the child and the skill of the anaesthetist.

All equipment necessary for an emergency intubation should be available with the suction controller turned on and a slight head-down tilt on the trolley. A rapid sequence induction technique is preferred by some anaesthetists with pre-oxygenation, thiopentone or propofol (in reduced dose), atropine, suxamethonium, and cricoid pressure. The child should be supine on the trolley for ease of induction and intubation unless the anaesthetist is familiar with intubation in the lateral position. Other anaesthetists use an inhalational technique with nitrous oxide, oxygen, and halothane intubating the child when deeply anaesthetized. The child should be extubated in the lateral position when awake.

Ear

Minor

Minor procedures are usually carried out as day cases and these include myringotomy and insertion of grommets for draining fluid in the middle ear. One of the major problems with these children is that of associated upper respiratory tract infections ('snuffly nose'). However, as long as the temperature is normal and there are no abnormal sounds in the chest on auscultation, surgery can proceed (see also Chapter 5).

Major

These include congenital defects of the ears associated with Treacher Collins syndrome and Goldenhar's syndrome. Mastoidectomy, myringoplasty, and tympanoplasty are uncommon operations in children now that ear infections are treated with antibiotics. Surgery for these procedures requires a careful anaesthetic technique since they are carried out using the operating microscope. Careful positioning of the child with head-up tilt, and avoiding anything that causes venous bleeding will give good operating conditions. Occasionally, induced hypotension will be required and those techniques used in adults can be employed. The agent of choice is probably labetalol in bolus doses of 0.2 mg kg^{-1} until the desired effect is achieved. This technique can be used without direct arterial monitoring (using an oscillometric technique).

Adrenalin may be used for infiltration and halothane should be avoided. A non-depolarizing muscle relaxant technique should be used with appropriate analgesics. Dizziness and sickness can be a difficult post-operative problem in any procedure involving the ear. Conventional anti-emetics may be given but repeat doses of dopamine-antagonists e.g. metoclopramide may lead to oculogyric crises. Ondansetron given in a single dose at operation (100 μg kg^{-1}) is a safe alternative.

Nose

Choanal atresia can be unilateral or bilateral and may be a membranous or bony obstruction of the nostril. Since neonates are obligatory nose-breathers, a bilateral obstruction can result in respiratory distress very rapidly and can only be relieved by taping an oral tube in the mouth and carrying out surgery as soon as possible. A stent is placed in the nostril and anaesthesia includes all the normal problems associated with neonatal surgery. The stent must remain *in situ* for about 6 weeks and there may be problems with blockage of the tube.

Endoscopy

The airway of small infants is very narrow and anything that reduces the diameter of the trachea will result in respiratory difficulties usually presenting as stridor. The function of the paediatric airway can be studied using straightforward chest and neck X-rays and if necessary new imaging techniques. Any external compression can usually be visualized using a barium swallow (e.g. vascular anomalies). CAT scans and MRI may be useful techniques prior to endoscopy (see pp. 203, 208).

Procedures used include

direct laryngoscopy
microlaryngoscopy
bronchoscopy
oesphagoscopy

Laryngoscopy/microlaryngoscopy

The predisposing problem with the airway may cause difficulties with induction of anaesthesia, and all sedative premedication should be avoided. Atropine should be given (10 μg kg^{-1}) because it will reduce secretions which will enhance the action of local anaesthetic drugs and reduce the requirement for regular suctioning of the airway.

Inhalation induction with oxygen and halothane is the technique of choice if there is pre-existing airway obstruction. In these cases it may be better to induce anaesthesia before attempting venous cannulation as stridor may be made worse if the child is stressed by the venepuncture. Induction may be prolonged but once an effective seal can be achieved with a mask, continuous positive airway pressure (CPAP) can be applied which will speed up induction. The child can be intubated using a deep volatile anaesthetic technique or, if the anaesthetist feels there is no difficulty with the airway, suxamethonium can be used. The trachea and larynx should be sprayed with lignocaine (maximum 4–5 mg kg^{-1}). Occasionally the child may already be intubated with a nasal tube and this may need to be changed to an oral tube.

The child's airway is then secure whilst the surgeon is preparing the equipment for the microlaryngoscopy. When everything is ready the endotracheal tube can be withdrawn and the anaesthetic can be continued using an insufflation technique with oxygen and halothane or increments of intravenous agent. A range of uncut endotracheal tubes must always be available in case of difficulties. If required an endotracheal tube can be passed into the trachea through the laryngoscope by the surgeon. Jet ventilation techniques are not recommended in smaller children but can be used for teenagers.

Laser surgery

This technique is now used for removal of lesions in the larynx, especially laryngeal papillomata. This condition usually involves multiple anaesthetics and management of the child can be very difficult. The initial problem is securing the airway as for microlaryngoscopy. However, there are several problems associated with the use of the laser.

1. A special endotracheal tube must be used, non-flammable, flexometallic.

2. The inspired oxygen concentration should be as near to 21% as possible to reduce the risk of fire. Adequate oxygen saturation must, however, be maintained.

3. The eyes of everyone in the operating theatre must be covered using goggles to protect against the laser beam.

Bronchoscopy

This is a procedure that is carried out less often in children than adults and is used as a diagnostic procedure, for removal of foreign bodies, and for removal of secretions (e.g. in cystic fibrosis). The airway is shared by both the anaesthetist and endoscopist and close co-operation is needed to ensure that the airway is not compromised. Anaesthetists often carry out broncho-scopies in intensive care units. In this case a second anaesthetist must be present to supervise and monitor the child. Modern ventilating broncho-scopes (e.g. Storz) can now be used in neonates. Preparation is the same as for laryngoscopy. Sedative premedication can be given if there is no risk of upper airway obstruction.

General anaesthesia is always used in children, sometimes combined with local analgesia. There is differing opinion on whether ventilation should be spontaneous or controlled, but this usually depends on the reason for bron-choscopy and the size of the child. Full monitoring is essential, with special emphasis placed on the capnograph. All children should be intubated first because this ensures that the anaesthetist knows the size of the endotracheal tube and in small infants this will determine the size of bronchoscope used.

Two types of bronchoscope are available. The Negus was originally a non-ventilating bronchoscope but one can employ the venturi principle to venti-late with oxygen-enriched air, whilst the child is kept asleep using intravenous drugs. The technique is only safe if the pipeline pressure (4.2 bar or approxi-mately 4200 kPa) can be adjusted and the appropriate injection needle is attached to the open lumen of the bronchoscope. This technique is only suit-able for older children (e.g. over 40 kg) as the needle size is critical and barotrauma can easily occur.

However, many centres now use the Storz ventilating bronchoscope (Fig. 8.2), with a Hopkins telescope to which a T-piece can be attached.

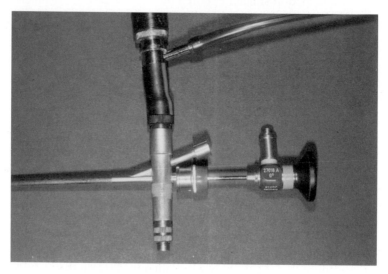

Fig. 8.2 Storz bronchoscope with T-piece attached.

and an analgesic infusion are essential. Two intravenous lines (one of which may be a central venous catheter) and an arterial line should be used, together with appropriate monitoring.

A hypotensive technique should be used unless cord monitoring is in progress but careful positioning can help to reduce blood loss. A simple hypotensive technique includes the use of labetalol and volatile agent, e.g. isoflurane. A hypotensive technique cannot be used with SSEP. The post-operative management includes good pain control using a continuous intra-venous analgesic infusion (perhaps patient-controlled analgesia, PCA, see p. 218), or epidural infusion via a catheter placed under direct vision by the surgeon. A nasogastric tube is advisable (gastric dilatation can occur), and a chest X-ray to exclude pneumothorax is desirable. The anaesthetic manage-ment described so far can be used for both a posterior approach to the spine, Harrington Rod instrumentation, or an anterior approach, Zilkie instrumen-tation or Dwyer's procedure. However, the anterior approach to the vertebral column is through the chest wall on the convex side of the curve, and this includes division of the diaphragm. This may result in more complications in the post-operative period which usually require admission to the intensive care unit for careful observation and in some cases a short period of post-operative ventilation.

PLASTIC SURGERY

These children can be divided into two groups. Firstly, those children with congenital deformities requiring surgery at a young age, and secondly, acquired problems as a result of trauma, burns etc. Both groups of chil-dren, depending on their age, may be psychologically upset by their deform-ity and need careful reassurance. It is also very important to remember that parents may be extremely stressed when their child is born with a complex facial deformity. There is a high incidence of associated anom-alies. Many deformities involving the head and neck also need careful assessment of their airway e.g. Pierre Robin syndrome and Treacher Collins syndrome (p. 122).

The general anaesthetic management of many children requiring plastic surgery, e.g. correction of 'bat ears', peripheral surgery for nerve and tendon repairs, or removal of peripheral lesions, is straightforward and can be combined with regional analgesic techniques where applicable. Bleeding can be a problem with removal of some lesions and this is often controlled by the surgeon using local infiltration and adrenalin 1 in 200 000. Care needs to be taken when halothane is employed but adrenalin can be safely used with the halogenated ethers. Full monitoring of these patients is always carried out.

However, some of these cases can be very demanding and their management will be discussed briefly in the next section.

Cleft lip and palate

Cleft lip can occur with or without a cleft palate and is one of the few congenital neonatal surgical problems that does not require early operation. The condition arises as a result of failure of fusion of the medial and lateral nasal swelling which normally is complete by the 7th week of fetal life. Occasionally this process fails and can result in a simple hare lip deformity or a complete bilateral cleft lip and palate. The condition, either simple or complex, occurs in approximately one in 600 of all births. Feeding problems may occur but if a cleft palate is present this can be helped by using a dental plate. The cleft lip is usually repaired between 8 and 12 weeks but it is believed by some surgeons that it would be beneficial to both the child and parents if the repair was carried out early in the neonatal child. Cleft palate repair is carried out at about 6 months. The management of the two conditions, although embryologically closely linked, is totally different. Cleft lip can often occur without any associated defect of the palate and without any other congenital abnormalities. On the other hand, an isolated cleft palate lesion is often associated with multiple congenital abnormalities, particularly congenital heart defects, which are recognized in typical syndromes (see below).

Cleft lip/palate without associated congenital abnormalities

It is essential to exclude any associated airway problems. If there is any evidence of an upper respiratory tract infection, then the procedure must be postponed. This can be a difficult decision since many children present with a runny nose, but they must be apyrexial with no chest signs. The anaesthetic management is uncomplicated, using a muscle-relaxant technique and a RAE endotracheal tube. A pack should be placed in the pharynx. If there is an associated cleft palate, the blade of the laryngoscope may disappear into the cleft. This can be avoided by using a gauze swab to cover the cleft.

Cleft palate with associated congenital abnormalities

If there is a solitary cleft palate, the condition is often associated with other congenital abnormalities, mainly involving the heart, jaw, and neck. The common syndromes seen are:

- Pierre Robin syndrome:
  cleft palate, micrognathia (which improves as the child grows) glossoptosis, occasional congenital heart disease (CHD);

lated. The incidence of vomiting is very high after squint surgery and this may be worsened by the administration of opioids which are not necessary in most younger children. The incidence of vomiting is significantly reduced by metoclopramide and ondansetron[7, 8] and by the use of propofol rather than thiopentone.

More stimulating procedures, such as evisceration for tumour, may require opioid analgesia or retrobulbar block. Whatever the anaesthetic technique chosen, it must include full vagal blockade with atropine or glycopyrronium to prevent the oculocardiac reflex.

Because of the nature of extra-ocular muscle, it does not behave in the same way as other striated muscle. The response to suxamethonium is one of sustained contraction which raises the IOP (which is not of consequence in this type of surgery) but more importantly restricts movement of the globe and may interfere with the surgeon's assessment of the squint (forced duction test). For this reason, if the patient is to breathe spontaneously, intubation under deep inhalational anaesthesia or following a short-acting non-depolarizing relaxant is preferable. If mivacurium is used together with inhalational anaesthesia, spontaneous ventilation returns within a few minutes of intubation.

NEUROSURGERY

Before embarking on any neurosurgical procedure, the important general principles of intracranial physiology must be understood. These include intracranial pressure (ICP) and the effects of any marked alterations in ICP, cerebral blood flow and its autoregulation, cerebral perfusion pressure, and cerebral venous pressure.

Intracranial pressure (ICP)

Contained within the skull are the brain, blood vessels, and cerebrospinal fluid. Any increase in the volume of any one component will generally result in a reduction of another. While the fontanelles and sutures are unfused in small infants, the skull does not act as a fixed volume container, thus allowing for some expansion which is not possible in an older child or adult.

Cerebral blood flow (CBF)

Autoregulation of the size of the cerebral vessels enables the blood flow to remain constant, irrespective of blood pressure fluctuations even as low as 45–50 mmHg in a supine infant. Hypercapnia causes vasodilatation with an increase in CBF and a rise in ICP. Cerebral vasoconstriction results from a low arterial carbon dioxide tension with a fall in CBF and ICP.

Cerebral perfusion pressure (CPP)

This is the difference between mean arterial blood pressure and the intracranial pressure.

Cerebral venous pressure

Any rise in intrathoracic pressure or central venous pressure will also result in an increase in ICP by increasing cerebral venous pressure.

CONTROL OF INTRACRANIAL PRESSURE

A detailed knowledge of the pharmacological effects that specific anaesthetic drugs exert on intracranial physiology is essential.

Ventilation

Positive end-expiratory pressure should be avoided because it will increase cerebral venous pressure. It is possible to maintain the $PaCO_2$ at 25 mmHg which will reduce the size of the brain with a lowering of the ICP by using modern ventilators and monitoring the end tidal carbon dioxide tension. It has been suggested that hyperoxia PaO_2 >150 mmHg) may have a beneficial effect in patients with gross cerebral oedema due to a greater tissue gradient,and this level should be maintained during surgery.[9] Good positioning of the patient is important to avoid any rise in venous pressure and a slight head-up tilt is beneficial.

Cerebral dehydration

Diuretics can be used to reduce both the intracellular and extracellular fluid volume. Frusemide in a dose of 0.5 mg kg^{-1} given after induction can be employed. Mannitol 20 per cent in a dose of 1–1.5 g kg^{-1}, again given immediately after induction, can also be used. Half is given over 10–20 min and the remainder slowly. The effect lasts 4–5 h but there is a danger of a rebound effect causing a rise in ICP due to the drug crossing the blood–brain barrier into the brain cells.

The urine volume must always be measured when diuretics are used. When the urine volume equals 10 per cent of the estimated blood volume, further urine losses must be replaced with Hartmann's solution.

Drugs

Steroids have been used to reduce cerebral oedema associated with tumours. They must be given pre-operatively and continued post-operatively.

Dexamethasone (0.25 mg kg^{-1} stat followed by 0.1 mg kg^{-1} every 6 h) is commonly used, and the dose is reduced over the next 7 days.

Hypotensive techniques

These techniques can be used in children. However, the blood pressure and heart rate should only be reduced to an appropriate level for the child. Labetalol (initial dose 0.5–1 mg kg^{-1}) can be used. When operating on vascular malformations it may be necessary to use sodium nitroprusside (0.3–1.5 μg kg^{-1} min^{-1}). However sodium nitroprusside does inhibit autoregulation and may result in a rise in ICP.

Anaesthetic drugs

The choice of drugs used depends on the effects that the individual drug has on cerebral function. Beneficial effects obviously include a reduction in ICP and maintenance of CPP. Also the drug ideally should not influence cerebrospinal fluid secretion or autoregulation.

Barbiturates

These drugs have many suitable features for neuro-anaesthesia, including a reduction in cerebral metabolism and blood flow with protection of autoregulation. These effects may be beneficial against ischaemic brain damage, together with useful anti-epileptic properties.

Propofol

Again cerebral flood flow and metabolism are diminished. However, dangerous falls in blood pressure on induction must be avoided. It has been used as a continuous intravenous infusion with an infusion of a short-acting analgesic drug such as alfentanil.

Opioids

These do not have any major effects on cerebral haemodynamics but should always be used with muscle relaxants to avoid muscular rigidity that can occur with, for example, large doses of fentanyl.

Volatile anaesthetics

Isoflurane is the drug of choice for maintenance and has been shown in those patients without intracranial pathology not to increase CBF and reduces cerebral metabolic rate (less than 1.5 minimal alveolar concentration).[10] Concentrations of up to 2% in air/oxygen are well tolerated.

Anaesthetic technique

Pre-operative assessment is important and must include neurological assessment of the child. Any signs of raised ICP will influence the anaesthetic technique adopted. All drugs that depress respiration or prolong recovery should be avoided. Occasionally a sedative premedicant drug is used in small children if the ICP is not raised. Atropine may be used for its antisialogogue effects because excessive saliva may compromise the airway. EMLA or amethocaine cream should be used for all children.

During induction of anaesthesia it is important to prevent the child from crying with a subsequent rise in ICP. Skilled venepuncture is possible with suitable pre-operative application of local anaesthetic cream followed by thiopentone and suxamethonium with lignocaine spray to the trachea. An armoured endotracheal tube should be used and a standard anaesthetic technique with moderate hyperventilation, non-depolarizing muscle relaxant, and analgesic can be used. The technique used should result in a rapid postoperative recovery. A stormy gaseous induction with halothane or other volatile agent may result in a rise in ICP and should be avoided. Isoflurane is useful as a maintenance agent because of the rapid recovery but is not an ideal induction agent for unpremedicated children.

Full monitoring should be used, with special emphasis on capnography. Temperature maintenance may be a problem during long procedures. Hypothermia can be overcome by warming inspired gases and intravenous infusions. However, care must be taken in avoiding hyperthermia which will increase cerebral metabolism. Blood loss needs careful measurement.

Post-operatively pain management is not a difficult problem but it is important to assess neurological function and carefully monitor respiratory status and fluid balance.

Neurosurgical problems

Specific problems that may be encountered are discussed briefly in this section following the guidelines already outlined.

Hydrocephalus

This is due to a blockage in the drainage of cerebrospinal fluid with resultant excessive accumulation of the fluid.

  Obstructive hydrocephalus
    Communicating: there is a clear communication to the subarachnoid space and it is often due to inflammatory changes.

Non-communicating: the obstruction is proximal to the subarachnoid space, e.g. Arnold–Chiari malformation or aqueduct stenosis.

Non-obstructive hydrocephalus.
This is due to a reduced size of brain substance or excessive production of cerebrospinal fluid.

Basically the operation carried out is a by-pass procedure to drain the excess fluid (shunt procedure). The drainage site may be the peritoneal cavity, the right atrium, occasionally to the pleural cavity, and very rarely to the 4th ventricle. The commonest shunt is the ventriculoperitoneal shunt because it allows for the growth of the child.

Problems may arise because the ICP may be very high and it might be necessary to tap off cerebrospinal fluid prior to surgery. No premedication is indicated and occasionally the procedure has to be carried out as an emergency. A standard anaesthetic for a neonate can be used.

Myelomeningocele

This condition occurs due to the lack of fusion of the neural tube in fetal life and an area of spinal canal is left without any bone cover (spina bifida). There is an associated neurological defect depending on the complexity of this lesion and this affects the sphincters and lower limbs. This condition is often associated with hydrocephalus.

Encephalocele

This is a defect involving the skull and brain. The problems encountered depend on the size of the malformation. Again this condition is often complicated by hydrocephalus.

The main problems encountered in both these conditions are related to the size of the lesion which may make it difficult to position the child for intubation.

Intracranial tumours

The central nervous system is one of the commonest sites for tumours in childhood, often located in the posterior cranial fossa. They may also cause hydrocephalus with a raised ICP by obstructing the outflow from the 3rd ventricle.

The operative procedure is a craniotomy. Again it is essential to avoid sedative opioid premedication. Posterior fossa surgery in the sitting position is technically more difficult because it can increase the risk of air embolism. This is not common if the prone position is adopted. The signs to look for are arrhythmias or changes in blood pressure during dissection around the hypothalamus or pituitary gland.

Haematoma — extradural or subdural

These may result from birth trauma and need operative treatment in the first 6–12 months of life.

Craniosynostosis

A condition in which premature closure of one or more sutures of the skull occurs. It is often associated with craniofacial abnormalities such as Crouzon's disease and Apert's syndrome. Early operative intervention gives better cosmetic results. However, if there is any sign of raised ICP, surgery may be necessary immediately.

DENTAL SURGERY

Children occasionally undergo in-patient surgery but more commonly dental surgery is carried out as an out-patient procedure. The former is carried out on children who have specific medical conditions, e.g. congenital heart disease, cystic fibrosis, mental retardation, etc., and their anaesthetic management is very similar to that used for an ENT operation, i.e. a shared airway with blood in the nasopharynx. The main difference is the requirement for a nasal airway rather than oral and the use of a pack in the oropharynx.

Out-patient surgery

The general principles of day case surgery apply but there are conditions specific to dental surgery that need to be considered.

- Children require anaesthesia more often than adults and they are usually uncooperative, having had previous extraction attempts using local analgesia.

- The children may be sleep-deprived due to pain from abscesses, they may be hungry, and basically just 'plain grizzly'.

- The dental pre-operative visit should screen out any difficult cases using a medical questionnaire and the children should all be ASA category 1 or 2.

- The preparation is not as simple as for day case hospital patients because the child is often brought in 10–15 min prior to treatment (i.e. 'just off the street') and the anaesthetist will not have the benefit of being able to use local anaesthetic cream or premedication if required.

- The usual conflicts arise when the airway is shared by two operators. However, many dental surgeons now work with the child in the supine position rather than the sitting position which was practised until recently.

- The skill of the anaesthetist is very important in dental anaesthesia and a careful induction, preferably with an indwelling cannula using propofol (3 mg kg^{-1}) is the technique of choice. The anaesthetic is continued with nitrous oxide, oxygen, and volatile agent, remembering that many of these children have had a previous anaesthetic. A nasal or laryngeal mask is used, and occasionally a nasopharyngeal airway will be required (beware adenoids in small children which may bleed). An upper respiratory tract infection with blockage of the nose would be a definite contraindication to surgery. Monitoring can be carried out with a pulse oximeter. The electrocardiogram is less often used. Recovery in the lateral position with slight head down tilt is essential because of blood in the airway. Checks must be carried out to ensure that no packs are left in the mouth. All blood loss should have stopped before the child is allowed home, preferably not using public transport.

REFERENCES

1. Haugen, D., Linker, D., Eik-Nes, S. *et al.* (1991). Congenital diaphragmatic hernia: determination of the optimal time for operation by echocardiagraphic monitoring of the pulmonary artery pressure. *Journal of Paediatric Surgery*, **26**, 560.
2. Walters, C. H. *et al.* (1988). Diclofenac sodium of post-tonsillectomy pain in children. *Anaesthesia*, **43**, 641.
3. Loughnan, B. A. and Fennelly, M. E. (1995). (Editorial) 1995 *Anaesthesia*, **50**, 101.
4. Hall, J. E., Levine, C. R., and Sudhir, K. G. (1978). Intraoperative awakening to monitor spinal cord function during Harrington instrumentation and spinal fusion. Description of procedures and report of three cases. *Journal of Bone and Joint Surgery*, **60**, A533.
5. Ausinsch, B. *et al.* (1975). Intraocular pressure in children during isoflurane and halothane anaesthesia. *Anesthesiology*, **42**, 167.
6. Brown, D. J., McGrand, J. A., and Palmer, J. R. (1976). Intraocular pressures after suxamethonium and endotracheal intubation in patients pre-treated with pancuronium. *British Journal of Anaesthesia*, **48**, 1201.
7. Bradman, L. M. *et al.* (1990). Metoclopramide reduces the incidence of vomiting following strabismus surgery in children. *Anesthesiology*, **72**, 245.
8. Rose, J. B., Martin, T. M., Corddry, D. H. *et al.* (1994). Ondansetron reduces the incidence and severity of poststrabismus repair vomiting in children. *Anesthesia Analgesia*, **79**, 486.
9. Swerdlow, D. B. (1983). Anaesthesia for neurosurgical procedures. In *Paediatric anaesthesia* Vol. 2 (ed. G. A. Gregory), pp. 679. Churchill Livingstone, New York.
10. Aligotsson, L. *et al.* (1988). Cerebral blood flow and oxygen consumption during isoflurane and halothane anaesthesia in man. *Acta Anaesthesiologica Scandinavica*, **32**, 15.

FURTHER READING

Gregory, G. A. (ed.) (1983). *Paediatric anesthesia,* Vols I and II. Churchill Livingstone, New York.

Smith, R. M. (ed.) (1980). *Anaesthesia for infants and small children.* C. V. Mosby, St Louis.

Steward, D. J. (1990). *Manual of pediatric anesthesia.* Churchill Livingstone, New York.

Sumner, E. and Hatch, D. J. (ed.) (1989). *Textbook of paediatric anaesthesia practice.* Bailliere Tindall, London.

Hughes, D. G., Mather, S. J., and Wolf, A. R. (eds). (1995). *Handbook of neonatal anaesthesia.* W. B. Saunders Co., London.

9

Day case anaesthesia

S. J. Mather

Operating upon children as day cases is not a new concept. As early as 1909 James Nicoll suggested such a possibility in the *British Medical Journal*. In 1985 the Royal College of Surgeons of England issued guidelines for day case surgery and these form the basis of operational policy for many units at the present time. Obviously not all procedures are suitable to be performed on a day stay basis, particularly those which result in more than transient or mild postoperative pain. Table 9.1 lists a variety of operations which are commonly performed as day cases.

SELECTION OF PATIENTS

The cost of day care surgery is, on average, considerably less than in-patient treatment of the same condition. This, in part, has been the stimulus to the recent upsurge in day case surgery, together with pressure from groups such as 'Action for sick children'. The age of the child is an important considera-tion when planning surgery. Many centres would be reluctant to discharge an infant of less than 3 months of age the same day, particularly if the social circumstances of the family were less than ideal.

Any child which has been born prematurely is considered by many to be at risk from post-operative apnoea, even if no opioids have been used although the exact period of risk remains a subject of debate.[1] Statistically most apnoea spells have occurred by the age of 44 weeks postconception. Children can be considered for day case surgery if they have no history of apnoea by 48 weeks postconceptual age. Although no association has been proven between these children and siblings who have succumbed to sudden infant death syndrome (SIDS), many parents are understandably very anxious about the effects of anaesthesia and surgery on another child in the family if there has been an infant death.

The psychological trauma of admission to hospital may be minimized by limiting the stay to the operative day; this is greatly helped if a parent can accompany the child and stay with him as much as possible, in the ward, in the anaesthetic room, and even in the recovery room if space permits. It has been stated that the risks of acquiring nosocomial infection in day care units is

Table 9.1 Suitable operations for day care surgery

General surgery
Herniotomy
Orchidopexy
Endoscopy or rectal biopsy; anal stretch
Tongue tie
Removal of small surface lesions, e.g. lipoma

ENT surgery
Myringotomy and insertion of grommets; some adenoidectomies
Examination under anaesthesia (including direct laryngoscopy but NOT bronchoscopy)

Ophthalmology
Lacrimal duct probing; strabismus correction (vomiting can be a problem)

Orthopaedics
Examination or manipulation under anaesthesia
Minor procedures such as excision of small exostoses, removal of wires, percutaneous tenotomies
Application of plaster of paris

Urology
Cystoscopy
Circumcision (with caudal or penile block)

Dental and oral surgery
Conservation
Forceps and surgical extraction
Excision of minor lesions

This list is by no means exhaustive but conveys an idea of the type of operation which is suitable.

reduced compared with in-patient admission[2] but there seem to be no recent studies of the modern hospital environment which prove this applies today.

The physical status of the patient is clearly important. Patients should be ASA 1 or 2 and any chronic disease, such as diabetes, must be well controlled. It would be wrong, however, to exclude some children with chronic but stable conditions because they are often more susceptible to psychological trauma and hospital infection. The parents of such children are often well versed in their child's condition and understand his needs perhaps better than the doctors and nurses. If the parents cannot co-operate fully in the post-operative care of the child or are unwilling for him to undergo day care surgery, they should not be pressurized to accept it. If they cannot cope, the child will suffer more than he would have done in hospital. Community nursing can play an important role in post-operative care.

Parents and children should be encouraged to visit the hospital ward prior to admission for surgery. They should also receive a booklet or information sheet concerning the starvation regime and details of routine post-operative management. It is advantageous in certain communities for this also to be printed in languages other than English. A pre-operative questionnaire for the parents to fill in saves much time in assessment of the child and may alert the anaesthetist or surgeon to the need for a special investigation such as a sickle test. A pre-operative questionnaire used in Bristol is shown in Table 9.2.

INVESTIGATIONS

It is not necessary to perform routine investigations on fit children just because they are to have a minor operation. Urinalysis and clinical examination of the chest and cardiovascular system should be performed in every case. Reliable estimations of blood pressure are difficult to obtain in children under 5 years because they frequently do not co-operate. Most would agree that routine haemoglobin estimation is unnecessary in the healthy child.

If the procedure warrants such investigation it is perhaps not suitable for day care surgery. Special investigations must be performed if indicated, e.g. sickle test.

If blood has to be taken from the child, the use of local anaesthetic cream (p. 87) can render this ordeal almost atraumatic.

Many hospitals now provide pre-assessment clinics where an anaesthetist can see and examine the child a week or two prior to surgery. Any relevant investigations can be ordered at that time, the procedure can be explained and any questions the parent or child may have can be answered.

PRE-OPERATIVE STARVATION

The usual rules for pre-operative fasting apply. It is only necessary to fast children for 4 h prior to anaesthesia, less for infants who have been given only clear fluids for a few hours (see p. 81)

Unfortunately, logistical factors sometimes result in a prolonged period of starvation. 'Nothing to drink after midnight' for a list starting at 0900 is bad enough in itself, but children starve from bedtime and this may be 1900 or 2000, resulting in a period without oral intake of about 14 h even if first on the list.[3] If the child does not drink immediately post-operatively, this period may be increased. Such problems may be difficult to address in the out-patient context but attention to such detail is important. It is sometimes preferable for the parent to wake the child in the early hours for a drink than to allow starvation periods in excess of 12 hours to occur. Children on afternoon lists are more fortunate, they usually get breakfast!

PRE-OPERATIVE ASSESSMENT QUESTIONNAIRE

(TO BE COMPLETED BY THE PARENT/GUARDIAN)

NAME .... AGE................................

PROPOSED OPERATION ....

(Please answer the following questions by circling YES or NO and add details where required).

1. Is your child allergic to anything? YES NO	8. Does your child have any loose/capped/crowned or false teeth? YES NO
Please specify	
2. Does he/she bring up phlegm from the chest:-	Has your child had or does he/she suffer from:
a) Now? YES NO	9. Heart trouble YES NO
b) At intervals during the year? YES NO	
3. Does his/her chest ever sound wheezy? YES NO	10. Chest trouble/asthma YES NO
	11. Liver disease/jaundice YES NO
4. Has your child a croupy cough now, or in the past? YES NO	12. Kidney disease YES NO
5. Was your child born prematurely? YES NO	13. Diabetes YES NO
If YES, how early	14. Bleeding tendencies YES NO
	15. Epilepsy/Convulsions YES NO
6. Are you/or is your child of Negro or Eastern Mediterranean origin? YES NO	16. Inherited disease of any kind? YES NO
If yes, has he/she had a Sickle cell test? YES NO	Specify ....
7. Have you/your child or any member of your family had a problem with an anaesthetic? YES NO	17. Recent immunisation (within 2 months) YES NO
	18. Anything else? YES NO

19. Is your child taking any medicines/tablets or injections? YES NO

Please specify ....

20. Has your child had previous operations/anaesthetics? YES NO

Please specify (with date of operation). ....

....

21. Has your child been in hospital for anything else? YES NO

If yes, why? ....

When? ....

22. Is there anything you would like to discuss with your anaesthetist? YES NO

....

SIGNATURE (Mother/Father) .... Date ....

Table 9.2

PREMEDICATION

It is now recognized that most children can be managed without sedative premedication provided that a sympathetic, reassuring approach is used.[4,5] Involving the parents fully and allaying their concerns will reassure the child and help to relieve his anxiety.

The recent advent of EMLA cream has made intravenous induction of anaesthesia much more pleasant but there are one or two problems with its use. The cream itself may render the veins less conspicuous and so it should be removed 5 min or so before venepuncture, perhaps just before the child leaves the theatre reception area or ward, if this is close by. This vasoconstriction does not occur with amethocaine cream. Sometimes the local anaesthetic cream does not result in complete analgesia, especially if it has not been in contact with the skin for a full hour. It is therefore important that one should explain this to the parent at the pre-operative visit and ask them not to tell the child 'it wont hurt now' — it may do, but hopefully not as much! It is better to say to the child that the 'scratch' will hardly hurt at all. Despite this view, some anaesthetists feel that premedication with sedative drugs is desirable, even for day cases.[6] Antihistamines such as trimeprazine are anti-emetics but also increase the pH of gastric juice.[7] Undoubtedly, some children are difficult to manage without sedation and one must then seriously question whether such a child is suitable for day case surgery. If sedative premedication is used, opioids should be avoided because these may increase nausea and vomiting.[8] The most effective medication may be night sedation, given at home the evening before or early that day if the child wakes and is fretful. This may be a particular problem in children having repeat procedures, especially if a previous induction has been stormy. Anticholinergic premedication is normally unnecessary and such drugs can be given with induction if required for the procedure.

ANAESTHETIC TECHNIQUES SUITABLE FOR DAY CASE SURGERY

Certain criteria must be fulfilled to consider the technique suitable. It should:

- cause minimal distress to the child and his parent, especially in those children who may require several anaesthetics;
- provide operating conditions which are as good as any 'in-patient' technique for the procedure being carried out;
- result in minimal post-operative sedation, nausea, and vomiting;
- provide good post-operative analgesia.

It is important to remember that the child will be going home. If the operation was painless, e.g. an examination under anaesthesia, the child may want to play outside or ride his bicycle. Parents must be advised that such activities are unwise until the next day, even if the child feels well, because co-ordination may be impaired for several hours. Day care surgery must remain as safe as if the child were to remain in hospital. It must be remembered that the parents may find even minor post-operative sequelae frightening and difficult to handle.

INDUCTION OF ANAESTHESIA

The particular technique used is a matter of individual choice. Many small children will tolerate an inhalational induction and certain older ones might prefer a 'mask' to 'the scratch'. It is important to discuss this with the child on the pre-operative visit, so that he has had time to consider the alternatives. Some anaesthetists have been accused of not taking the child's feelings into account. It has to be said, however, that some children prefer not to have an anaesthetic at all and will agree to neither the 'scratch' nor the 'mask'. In these circumstances, an intravenous induction, skilfully performed while the parent distracts the child, is undoubtedly best. One should not persist, however, with difficult venepunctures if success seems remote.

For the child, these few moments before induction constitute what he will remember as 'his anaesthetic'. They can be the most psychologically damaging, more so even than post-operative pain. It is vitally important therefore that the situation is handled with skill and care.

Overall, propofol is probably the most widely used induction agent for day cases in the UK, but in small children the slight pain of injection may cause a withdrawal response of flexing the wrist, pulling the needle or cannula out of the vein. Firm restraint of the wrist and hand before injection is therefore essential and it is preferable to test for extravasation by injection of saline. Mixing lignocaine with the propofol is acceptable (see p. 24), even in small children. Many anaesthetists still use thiopentone for paediatric day cases because the smoothness of induction is unrivalled. Small doses may be used to precede application of the facemask as soon as consciousness is obtunded, induction being completed with a volatile agent. This reduces the hangover effect of the barbiturate. In any event, some practitioners consider that mild sedation following the procedure is beneficial. The use of thiopentone does not seem to significantly affect clinical recovery or delay discharge.

Other agents are, of course, available but offer no significant advantages. Ketamine would be considered by many to be unsuitable for day surgery because of its prolonged recovery characteristics and possible dysphoria. It is sometimes used, however, for brief but painful procedures such as bone marrow trephine in oncology cases.

MAINTENANCE OF ANAESTHESIA

It is preferable to use agents which are rapidly metabolized or excreted unchanged. For this reason inhalational techniques are most suitable, supplemented by small doses of a short-acting opioid such as alfentanil if required. By far the best supplementation is provided by local nerve blocks if these are feasible. Some sort of nerve block or infiltration can be provided for all the general surgical, orthopaedic, urological, and dental operations in Table 9.1 which will require post-operative analgesia (see Chapter 11). Ophthalmic surgery and insertion of grommets require little or no analgesia and can be managed with paracetamol.

The relative merits of the various inhalational agents are discussed elsewhere in this book but for practical purposes halothane is most suitable for inhalational induction of anaesthesia in unpremedicated patients. A sequential technique can be employed whereby another volatile agent is substituted for halothane once induction is complete. The very real risk of larynogspasm with isoflurane far outweighs the remote risk of halothane-associated hepatitis in this group of patients. If he is unpremedicated, the 'wet', frightened child is a daunting prospect for an isoflurane induction, even in expert hands.

On the whole it is desirable to avoid intubation if the child is going home the same day in case postintubation laryngeal oedema should develop. This, however, is a rare occurrence and provided the child is kept in hospital for 4 h it should be recognized and safety will not be compromised. Gentle laryngoscopy and selection of the correct size of tube will do much to minimize laryngeal oedema post-operatively.

If the child must be intubated for the procedure, deep halothane anaesthesia may avoid the need for muscle relaxants, particularly suxamethonium which is associated with muscle pain in the ambulatory patient. Such pain, however, is reported to be less in children.[9] Intubation under isoflurane and particularly enflurane is more difficult and may result in laryngospasm. Mivacurium is a suitable and preferable alternative to suxamethonium in the non-emergency patient. 100–150 μg kg^{-1} in combination with a volatile agent provides good intubating conditions. Spontaneous ventilation returns within 5–7 minutes and can be 'assisted' until the tidal volume is adequate. Apnoea following 10 μg kg^{-1} of alfentanil frequently lasts longer and this drug is commonly used in such doses for day cases. The laryngeal mask airway may have a particular niche in procedures involving the head and neck where the patient does not need to be intubated to allow the procedure to take place but access for the anaesthetist is restricted.

MONITORING DURING DAY CARE ANAESTHESIA

In most hospitals, day care surgery is performed in an operating theatre suite and as such it should be fully equipped for monitoring as outlined in Chapter

4. Certain situations, however, such as dental out-patient clinics may be less well equipped. A pulse oximeter must be considered the absolute minimum provision in such clinics. Non-invasive blood pressure monitoring may be useful but many procedures are too short to make such measurements feasible in practice. The average patient in a day care theatre suite will have electrocardiogram, blood pressure, and oxygen saturation monitored.

FLUID REGIMES

Under normal circumstances prolonged pre-operative starvation will not have occurred. Only rarely does the surgical procedure warrant intra-operative fluid administration but babies and small infants may benefit from intravenous maintenance fluid until they are able to drink. If this is not done the total peri-operative starvation period may be excessive and the incidence of nausea and vomiting is increased.

RECOVERY FROM ANAESTHESIA

Post-operatively the child should be cared for in a fully equipped recovery room staffed by trained nurses with the skill to manage the unconscious patient. As for in-patient surgery, oxygen should be given until the child is awake,[10] and requirements for day case anaesthesia are no different from those of in-patients. The child should be returned to his parents in the ward as soon as it is considered safe for him to leave the recovery room. This will greatly assist in comforting the child and should not be many minutes after leaving the theatre. In some hospitals it is feasible for the parent to collect the child from the recovery room door once he or she has awakened and reflexes have returned.

POST-OPERATIVE ANALGESIA

Since some procedures carried out as day cases will result in post-operative pain it is vital that attention is paid to achieving good post-operative analgesia. Once the child has left the hospital one is totally dependent on the parents to provide for the child's comfort. Clear instructions are therefore necessary and discussion with the parents should include an explanation of the likely sequelae to anaesthesia. One should mention the possibility of loss of appetite and nausea, which are common. One should point out that vomiting may occur at home and if it is prolonged they should telephone for advice. If a community nurse is available to visit the child on his return home, this will reassure the parents and will also provide the means by which the hospital can be quickly and reliably informed of any problems.

The use of nerve blocks greatly reduces the incidence of post-operative nausea and vomiting over that seen with opioid analgesia. The usual analgesic regimen advised when the child leaves hospital will be oral paracetamol 15 mg kg^{-1} 4 hourly up to 4 times daily possibly with non-steroidal anti-inflammatory analgesia in addition, e.g. diclofenac. It must not be forgotten, however, that opioids administered as part of the technique may result in the child being nauseated later[11] and he or she may not feel able to take the paracetamol orally. Nausea is very common after even minor surgery in children. Ibuprofen may be more potent than paracetamol and diclofenac has the advantage that it can be given rectally.[12]

If nausea and vomiting are prolonged, the child should be kept in hospital overnight. Dehydration can occur and must be avoided.

In such cases, parenteral fluid may be given overnight. No child who has been unable to drink clear fluids should be discharged home.

REFERENCES

1. Malviya, S., Swartz, J., and Lerman, J. (1993). Are all preterm infants younger than 60 weeks postconceptual age at risk for postanesthetic apnea? *Anesthesiology*, **78**, 1076.
2. Otherson, A. B. and Clatworth, H. W. (1968). Outpatient herniorrhapy for children. *American Journal of Diseases of Children*, **116**, 78.
3. Miller, D. C. (1990). Editorial. Why are children starved? *British Journal of Anaesthesia*, **64**, 4.
4. Beeby, D. G. and Morgan-Hughes, J. O. (1980). Behaviour of unsedated children in the anaesthetic room. *British Journal of Anaesthesia*, **52**, 297.
5. Steward, D. J. (1980). Anaesthesia for paediatric outpatients. *Canadian Anaesthetists Society Journal*, **27**, 412.
6. Brzustowixz, R. M. *et al.* (1984). Efficacy of oral premedication for paediatric outpatient surgery. *Anesthesiology*, **60**, 475.
7. Meakin, G., Dingwall, A. E., and Addison, G. M. (1987). Effects of fasting and oral premedication on the pH and volume of gastric aspirate in children. *British Journal of Anaesthesia*, **59**, 678.
8. Booker, P. D. and Chapman, D. J. (1979). Premedication in children undergoing day-care surgery. *British Journal of Anaesthesia*, **51**, 1083.
9. Bush, G. H. and Roth, F. (1961). Muscle pains after suxamethonium chloride in children. *British Journal of Anaesthesia*, **33**, 151.
10. Motoyama, E. K. and Glazener, C. H. (1986). Hypoxaemia after general anaesthesia in children. *Anesthesia and Analgesia*, **65**, 267.
11. Mather, S. J. and Peutrell, J. M. (1995). Post-operative morphine requirements following anaesthesia for tonsillectomy: comparison of intravenous morphine and non-opioid analgesic techniques. *Paediatric Anaesthesia*, **5**, 185–88.
12. Bone, M. E. and Fell, D. (1988). A comparison of rectal diclofenac with intramuscular papaveretum or placebo for pain relief following tonsillectomy. *Anaesthesia*, **43**, 277.

10

Anaesthesia for radiological procedures

J. W. O'Higgins

INTRODUCTION

An anaesthetist may be required to assist in the treatment of children under-going the following sophisticated procedures within specialized areas of a Radiology Department:

- computerized axial tomogram (CT) scanning;
- neuroradiological investigations;
- cardiac catheterization;
- bronchography
- other techniques — arteriography, venography, sialography, lithotripsy;
- radio-isotope scanning;
- magnetic resonance imaging (MRI).

Sedation may be acceptable to older children undergoing the above proce-dures. However, the provision of anaesthesia is necessary for many children under the age of 5 years, and some over that age, because they may not be able to lie perfectly still during the investigation which may be frightening, prolonged, uncomfortable, painful, and carried out on a hard table in unfa-miliar surroundings where parental presence may not be desirable. The anaesthetist's prime responsibility will be to ensure the patient's comfort and safety, to treat untoward events caused by drugs, contrast media, or other noxious stimuli, and to maintain cardiorespiratory stability. The anaesthetist is time- and cost-effective because he should be able to guarantee a safe, still patient, allowing good film quality for accurate diagnosis and therefore no need to repeat the investigation.

THE CHANGING PATTERN OF RADIOLOGICAL PRACTICE

During the last 25 years, there has been a profound change in the type and frequency of anaesthetic-associated radiological investigations. The number of air-encephalograms (AEG), myelograms, and bronchograms have decreased dramatically so that these procedures are seldom performed at the present time in Britain. Their place has been taken in most instances by the introduction into clinical practice of the ultrasound scanner, the CT scanner in the 1970s and MRI in the 1980s. Similarly, the role of cardiac catheterization in the investigation and diagnosis of congenital heart disease has altered since the widespread use of two-dimensional echocardiography during the last 20 years. As a consequence there are fewer children catheterized today. Carotid angiography, too, has changed from a threatening procedure requiring an injection into a major neck vessel into a less traumatic one involving femoral arterial puncture. There has, then, been a shift from the invasive to the non-invasive, or minimally invasive, diagnostic procedures.

Recent developments in cardiology in the field of therapeutic interventional techniques have added a further dimension to catheterization, and have made the presence of the anaesthetist more essential than previously.

Major changes have taken place in the clinical composition of the contrast media used in so many of these procedures. In 1968, the introduction of the first non-ionic, low-osmolality intravenous contrast medium heralded a new era of patient-friendly, less toxic agents, thereby decreasing the side-effects and risks of the investigations.

Changes in anaesthetic agents, relaxants, and monitoring have also played a role in the advances made in patient care during the same period.

GENERAL CONSIDERATIONS

The environment

Certain features of the Radiology Department and its equipment are less than ideal for the administration of anaesthesia.
These features are:

- the location
- the X-ray room
- equipment
- anaesthetic assistance
- the radiographer.

The location

Most X-ray departments are situated some distance away from operating theatres, intensive care units, and other areas which are well-frequented by anaesthetists. Unless they have regular sessions in the department, the anaesthetists are occasional visitors and are probably unfamiliar with its layout. These factors may cause uncertainty and difficulties for them, particularly in emergency situations, and may mean that a second anaesthetist is seldom immediately available should the first one require urgent help. As a consequence, only well-trained, experienced anaesthetists should be asked to work in these departments.

The X-ray room

The anaesthetist is often required to work in a small, cramped, uncomfortable space and with difficult access to his patient due to the close proximity of the radiological apparatus. The room may be darkened and the patient covered by sterile towels, thus making clinical observation difficult. This difficulty is exacerbated by the need for the anaesthetist to be some distance from the patient when the X-rays are taken.

Most X-ray rooms are kept cool so that the sophisticated electrical and electronic equipment works efficiently. Babies and small children need to be kept warm, so the anaesthetist may have to insist on a high ambient temperature and the provision of gamgee, blankets, and other aids to maintain normothermia.

Equipment

Anaesthetic equipment must be checked thoroughly before induction of anaesthesia, because duplicates may not be readily available or close at hand — there is no second theatre nearby. Monitoring equipment is essential and requires regular maintenance and checking. It is liable to malfunction and breakage if it is moved frequently in and out of X-ray rooms.

Piped gases may not be available in every area so the anaesthetist must remember to check his cylinders regularly, even though he may be out of the habit of doing so. Suction apparatus must be checked, particularly as X-ray tables may not tilt adequately or fast enough.

Anaesthetic assistance

An anaesthetic nurse or operating department assistant is seldom permanently attached to the Radiology Department. Nevertheless the anaesthetist must insist on trained assistance in this area. The assistant should be given time to become acquainted with the layout, supply of drugs, gases, suction, and emergency apparatus before the induction of anaesthesia. A radiological nurse may be more familiar with the environment but she is unlikely to be trained to assist the anaesthetist adequately.

The radiographer

The radiographer should be reminded of the need for the anaesthetist to be informed before the patient is moved suddenly, contrast medium is injected, or radiographs are taken.

Pre-investigation care

All children requiring anaesthesia must be adequately assessed beforehand. Potential problems may relate to:

- transport
- temperature
- pre-investigation feeding
- premedication

Transport

Small, often very sick children may have to be transported long distances to specialized centres, usually by ambulance and often with experienced medical and nursing personnel.

Temperature

It is essential that these infants be kept in the best condition and that they do not become cold. Radiant lamps, incubators, blankets, hats, and bootees may be necessary.

Pre-investigation feeding

Small infants may need intravenous glucose before and during the investigation if there is danger of hypoglycaemia.

Premedication

Premedication is contraindicated for children with cerebral trauma, raised intracranial pressure, respiratory difficulty, and those who have a long journey to reach the radiology department. Analgesics and respiratory depressants should be avoided. Mild hypnotics may be suitable, together with topical local anaesthetic cream. Phenothiazines may be given to reduce the side-effects of contrast media, but they may cause cardiovascular changes and respiratory embarrassment in sensitive patients.

Irradiation

The patient

Children should be given maximal protection against overexposure to irradiation. No known level of ionizing irradiation is totally safe. The effects of irradiation to young children are greater than those to older persons, particularly when considering exposure to gonads, active bone marrow, and the thyroid gland. Special lead/protective shields should be used whenever possible. Technological advances have reduced both scatter and exposure times. The anaesthetist can contribute by providing excellent conditions and immobility so that repeat films become unnecessary, and irradiation is kept to a minimum. Cardiac catheterization, in particular, is known to be associated with high absorbed thoracic X-ray dosage,[1] and the procedure is frequently repeated on the same patient.

The anaesthetist

The anaesthetist, and particularly onc who has a regular session in the department, should be aware of the dangers to which he is exposed. He should wear protective clothing, even though it is heavy, hot, and cumbersome. Lead coats may protect gonads but seldom cover the thyroid gland. Lead gloves impair manual dexterity, so elective intubation or the use of a laryngeal mask is safer than holding a face mask on a patient with a difficult airway. Gloves also render it impossible to feel the pulse, so that if they are worn, greater reliance must be placed on monitoring.

The anaesthetist's dilemma is to observe the patient closely, yet not expose himself to excessive radiation. He will reduce his own risk by distancing himself from the source of the irradiation but this usually means standing far away from the patient. In these circumstances, adequate monitoring and extra vigilance are vital for patient safety. Circumstances may dictate that the anaesthetist leave the room during a period of heavy exposure, and in these circumstances the monitors must be visible to the anaesthetist through a glass window, or on closed circuit television screens.

It should be noted that irradiation is not involved in patients undergoing MRI.

Contrast media

Contrast media are frequently injected into children during radiological procedures in order to delineate blood vessels, CSF spaces, airways, urinary tracts, the gut, and other areas. They are based on benzene-ring compounds, with iodine atoms attached.

Side-effects and reactions associated with intravascular contrast media are related to:

- hyperosmolality
- ionization
- anaphylactoid responses
- volume and speed of injection

Hyperosmolality

Virtually all contrast media are hyperosmolar (300–2200 mosmol l^{-1}). When hyperosmolar solutions are injected intravascularly, they cause:

- a rapid increase in blood volume, at the expense of an initial interstitial and intracellular dehydration, which is followed by the later onset of an osmotic diuresis and generalized dehydration; the rise in blood volume may cause ventricular arrhythmias, an increase in ventricular workload, and cardiac decompensation which may be in part related to increased calcium binding;

- vasodilatation, with flushing of the skin;
- damage to endothelial cells, leading to thrombophlebitis;
- red blood cell deformation, particularly significant in children with sickle-cell disease, who may develop tissue hypoxia;
- capillary damage, causing tissue oedema.

Related symptoms include nausea and vomiting, pain, discomfort, and a feeling of warmth. The patient may cough if the agent is injected into the right ventricle. All these symptoms are greatly reduced in frequency and intensity if non-ionic contrast media are used.

The development 25 year ago of non-ionic low osmolar (300–700 mosmol l^{-1}) contrast media has been associated with the concomitant reduction in side-effects and reactions when compared with the earlier ionic, high osmolar (1500–2200 mosmol l^{-1}) agents. The advantages of the more modern, patient-friendly products are sufficient to outweigh the disadvantage of the fivefold increase in cost.

Ionization

The early contrast agents were ionized molecules which had a very high osmolality but which also contained free sodium ions. These ions caused a rise in serum sodium levels, with the consequent risk of precipitating pulmonary oedema, cerebral oedema, renal failure, and poor ventricular function. Recently developed agents are non-ionic and consequently safer.

Anaphylactoid responses

Adverse reactions to contrast media occur in 5–8 per cent of patients injected, and they range from itching and urticaria to full-blown anaphylactoid reactions with bronchospasm and cardiovascular collapse. The mortality from the intravascular administration of these agents is approximately one in 40 000 patients. Pretreatment with steroids in high-risk patients might reduce this incidence.[2]

Volume and speed of injection

The increase in blood volume following the intravascular administration of contrast will be related to the volume injected. It is recommended that no more that 1 ml of contrast medium per kg body weight should be given intravenously to any patient as a bolus, and that this volume should not be repeated for at least 10 min. A maximum of 4 ml kg^{-1} is allowed during one investigation. These recommendations aim to reduce the risk of fluid and electrolyte disturbances.

Monitoring

Careful and meticulous clinical observation, together with adequate, accurate monitoring is essential to ensure patient safety during and after anaesthesia. This statement is particularly true in the radiology department especially when the situation involves an unfamiliar, poorly-lit environment, limited access to the patient, and the anaesthetist often some distance from the patient. Essential monitoring includes the following:

- Pulse oximeter
- ECG
- Non-invasive blood pressure
- Ventilator disconnection alarm
- Ventilator pressure
- Core temperature
- Capnography
- Inspired oxygen analyser.

Closed circuit television may also be necessary.

Post-investigation care

Children recovering from anaesthesia require adequate observation in a properly equipped recovery room with trained staff. If, as is often the case, such facilities are not available within the radiology department, the anaesthetist must ensure that the transfer to a suitable adjacent recovery area is undertaken safely.

Routine anaesthetic observations and treatment are required along with the following special considerations.

- Care must be taken to maintain a satisfactory fluid balance in children who have been given contrast media, which causes initial hypervolaemia and, later, cellular dehydration and a marked diuresis.
- Large cannulae may have been inserted into veins or arteries, so frequent assessment of the puncture sites are necessary to detect bleeding, haematoma formation, or decreased limb blood flow.
- Neurological observations may be required to safeguard children who have had intracranial investigations.
- Physiotherapy is needed after bronchography, to remove contrast medium from the lungs.
- Small children may need to be warmed to regain their normal temperature.

SPECIFIC PROCEDURES

CT scanning

This procedure is frequently used to investigate lesions throughout the body and it has markedly reduced the number of other radiological procedures undertaken. CT scanning is painless but it may be frightening to young children. In certain circumstances, parents may stay close to their children to give support and encourage co-operation. Children must remain perfectly still throughout the procedure, which may last for 10–40 min. Occasionally, diaphragmatic immobility is requested for periods of up to 10 s at a time. Frequent, noisy table movements often disturb sedated children. A bolus injection of approximately 1.5 ml kg^{-1} of contrast medium may be required before or during the investigation. Children with raised intracranial pressure, cerebral trauma, respiratory problems, or cardiovascular instability pose difficult problems for the anaesthetist.

Neonates frequently require no medication because they may sleep throughout the procedure. However, infants and children up to the age of 5 years usually require sedation or anaesthesia because they are unable or unwilling to co-operate sufficiently.

Numerous sedation regimes, using either oral, intravenous or intramuscular medications have been described,[3–5] but all suffer from the difficulty of predicting the exact dose requirement to ensure immobility without under- or overdosage. Moreover, excessive secretions, enlarged tonsils, and unsuspected hydrocephalus may cause problems.

Thompson suggested that general anaesthesia with endotracheal intubation is the technique of choice to ensure patient safety, excellent film quality, and efficient use of an expensive resource.[4] Approximately two-thirds of his patients under the age of 10 years were anaesthetized for the procedure.

When general anaesthesia is required the premedication, if any, should not cause respiratory depression and the induction agents must be short-acting. Triclofos premedication in non-neurological cases and an inhalational or propofol induction, followed by vecuronium, endotracheal intubation, and controlled mechanical ventilation with a nitrous oxide–oxygen mixture is suitable. Low doses of volatile agents may be added as required. Plastic endotracheal tube connections are routinely used nowadays but metal connectors are still in use in some hospitals, especially in sites where anaesthesia is infrequently given. Metal connectors should be avoided for CT scans because they can distort the image. The technique aims to achieve patient safety and comfort, good radiological conditions, and minimal post-anaesthetic depression — an important consideration when recovery facilities are less than optimal. Careful patient observation is supplemented by monitoring as outlined above.

Neuroradiological investigations

Sedative and anaesthetic techniques for neuroradiological procedures should ensure the provision of normal blood gases while at the same time avoiding fluctuations in arterial blood pressure. They should also permit assessment of the child's neurological state during and immediately after the investigation. Coughing and straining must be avoided and the hypertensive response to intubation should be attenuated.

CT scan of brain

Walters reported a 3–4 per cent need for anaesthesia amongst 5000 adult and paediatric patients undergoing CT scan in a British neurosurgical centre.[6] He maintains that most children do not require sedation or anaesthesia, but that in the uncooperative child, anaesthesia is essential.

Sedative techniques may be used on occasion provided that intracranial pressure is normal, but careful monitoring and a readiness to ensure adequate ventilation are essential. However, it is generally safer to anaesthetize than to sedate for this procedure.

Anaesthesia for CT scanning of the brain in children follows a similar pattern to that described for CT scanning above, but special consideration must be given to the risk of intracranial decompensation and possible raised intracranial pressure. Walters uses a light anaesthetic technique with controlled ventilation and minimal isoflurane.[6] He points out that unconscious patients undergoing a scan need the presence of an anaesthetist to ensure airway safety and respiratory adequacy. A rapid return to full consciousness is also important, as Wright states that in a survey of British neuroradiological units, only 30 per cent report adequate areas for the induction and recovery of anaesthetized patients.[7]

Cerebral angiography

Cerebral angiography is performed to investigate vascular and other lesions in the brain. Contrast medium is injected into the carotid or vertebral arteries either directly through the neck (seldom by this route nowadays), or more recently through a catheter introduced into the femoral artery and advanced cranially. The procedure is invasive and unpleasant, with severe headache and flushing of the skin as the contrast is injected. Virtually all cerebral angiography in children takes place under general anaesthesia, with intubation and moderate hyperventilation. The advantages of this method include patient comfort and safety, absence of movement, with a consequent reduction in the risk of haematoma formation or dissection at the vessel puncture site, and reduction in intracranial pressure. Hyperventilation has been reported to enhance film quality.

Air encephalography (AEG)

Air encephalography is now almost of historic interest, this investigation having been virtually replaced by the less invasive CT scan, but is included here for completeness. The technique is contraindicated in patients with raised intracranial pressure. The procedure involves a lumbar puncture and the injection of air into the cerebrospinal fluid. The air floats into the ventricles with the patient in the sitting position. A series of radiographs are then taken with the patient strapped securely into a chair and placed in different positions to outline various areas of the subarachnoid space and ventricles. The patient usually suffers from a severe headache and intense nausea afterwards. General anaesthesia with endotracheal intubation using an armoured tube is advisable. The anaesthetist must be prepared to deal with the potential occurrence of the following major problems:

- Hypotension in the sitting position in the anaesthetized child.

- Endotracheal tube obstruction, disconnection, or accidental extubation with disastrous consequences as the head and trunk are moved into various positions by persons unaware of the potential dangers of such movement.

- Damage to peripheral nerves by pressure in abnormal positions.

- The harness holding the head becoming too tight, thereby causing cerebral hypoperfusion and raised intracranial venous pressure.

- The rapid diffusion of nitrous oxide into the injected air in the ventricles, thereby increasing the size of the gas bubble and consequently causing a rise in intracranial pressure. The use of an oxygen/air mixture overcomes this.

- The sudden occurrence of respiratory depression, irregular breathing, and apnoea in the spontaneously breathing child with raised intracranial pressure.

The anaesthetic technique must ensure an adequate blood pressure to perfuse the brain in the sitting position, a clear airway, and adequate gas exchange. Controlled ventilation with muscle relaxation reduces the incidence of raised intracranial pressure but increases the problems if accidental extubation occurs. Spontaneous ventilation is not recommended, although it may give an indication of a high intracranial pressure when the respiratory pattern alters.

Monitoring must incorporate electrocardiography, blood-pressure measurement, capnography, and oximetry, whilst clinical observation should include palpation of the arteries above the neck and observation of the pupils. An ECG may demonstrate arrhythmias when air is injected into the cerebrospinal fluid space.

Myelography, radiculography, contrast ventriculography

These procedures are undertaken to delineate tumours, disc lesions, and other abnormalities in the spinal canal and the ventricles. The techniques involve the injection of contrast medium into the cerebrospinal fluid space and then a repositioning of the patient to demonstrate the suspected lesion. Ventriculography requires the same positions as for the AEG techniques, while myelography demands that the patient is tipped head up and head down so that the contrast moves throughout the cerebrospinal fluid space.

General anaesthesia is required when children are exposed to these studies, but the procedures are not as unpleasant or as hazardous as the AEG. Hypotension may occur when the patient is tilted head up. Phenothiazines may precipitate seizures in patients who have had subarachnoid metrizamide (Amipaque), but this contrast medium has been superseded by iohexol (Omnipaque) which carries far less risk.

Cardiac catheterization

Approximately 5000 children with congenital heart disease undergo cardiac catheterization each year in Britain, usually after the initial diagnosis has been made by echocardiography. Catheterization is undertaken both to confirm the anatomical diagnosis and to assess the shunts and pressures within the heart prior to cardiac surgery. Over 40 per cent of these children are below the age of 1 year, and most of them have complex lesions. Many are very ill, with a metabolic acidosis, hypoxaemia, congestive failure, and perhaps on anti-failure therapy.

In children, the catheter is inserted percutaneously through a femoral vein into the right heart chambers. If left heart catheterization is necessary, access may be across a patent foramen ovale, through a septal defect, trans-septally, or through a puncture site in a femoral artery. Angiography is usually performed with contrast medium at the end of the procedure.

Approximately 54 per cent of infants and children undergoing catheterization in Britain are sedated throughout the procedure, while the remainder are anaesthetized. Neonates are either anaesthetized, sedated, or given solely local anaesthesia in roughly equal numbers. whichever technique is used, it is essential to maintain cardiovascular stability, an unchanged inspired oxygen fraction, and near-normal, stable carbon dioxide levels while serial blood sampling is undertaken, so that the samples are genuinely comparable. Moreover, all children catheterized in the same hospital should be given the same anaesthetic or sedative technique, so that the cardiologist can compare the results between different children meaningfully.

If sedation is to be the technique of choice, it is usually prescribed by the cardiologist, and the anaesthetist attends only if an emergency occurs. The Toronto mixture of intramuscular pethidine, promethazine, and chlorpromazine is sometimes used, as are benzodiazepines, phenothiazines, barbiturates, and neuroleptic drugs. A sedative technique appears simple but suffers from the difficulty of forecasting the correct dose of drug for each individual patient. Overdose causes cardiorespiratory depression and increased pulmonary artery pressure, while underdosage leads to unstable and unsatisfactory conditions.

The author favours an anaesthetic technique which includes an oral hypnotic premedication followed by induction, muscle relaxation, intubation and controlled ventilation with nitrous oxide in 33 per cent oxygen. While it may be argued that such ventilation is unphysiological, the technique is inherently safe and it produces stable, reproducible conditions.

Whichever technique is used, adequate monitoring is essential. Complications which may occur during the procedure include arrhythmias, bleeding, infection, accidental perforation of the heart or great vessels, fluid imbalance, air embolism, hypoglycaemia, hypothermia, and problems associated with contrast media and the catheter itself.

Intervention techniques

Rashkind described balloon atrial septostomy as long ago as 1966, but during the last 10 years there has been a rapid increase in the number of children who have undergone other therapeutic procedures associated with catheterization. These procedures include balloon angioplasty and valvuloplasty, embolization, and the insertion of apparatus to close a patent ductus arteriosus. These techniques are hazardous, complicated, and frequently protracted. General anaesthesia is definitely indicated, with intubation and ventilation. Monitoring may include direct arterial pressure measurement. Resuscitation drugs and equipment must be close at hand.

Bronchography

There has been a decline in the use of bronchography in Britain since bronchiectasis and tuberculosis have become less common. Bronchiectatic children who need a bronchogram are frequently hypoxaemic and may produce copious thick sputum. They usually need physiotherapy and postural drainage for 1 or 2 days prior to the investigation.

Bronchography in children is carried out under general anaesthesia. Premedication may include an antisialogogue, while induction is followed by endotracheal intubation. The anaesthetist must be prepared to overcome bronchospasm caused by secretions, contrast medium, or the tube irritating a sensitized tracheal mucosa. Maintenance is usually provided by oxygen with minimal volatile or intravenous agents. Ventilation may be assisted or controlled.

Oily propyliodone is usually introduced directly by a catheter into one main bronchus and is encouraged to flow distally down the bronchi and bronchioles by the application of positive pressure ventilation. Radiographs are taken with the child's lungs held in full inspiration. The process is repeated in the other lung provided that the child's condition allows it. Oximetry is essential, both during and after the investigation.

After the radiography has been completed, as much of the contrast as possible is removed by suction and physiotherapy prior to extubating and awakening the child. Further physiotherapy is required, together with humidified oxygen, for several hours after the procedure, to reduce the incidence of post-investigation hypoxaemia.

Other techniques

Portocavograms, arteriograms, lymphangiograms, sialograms, and genito-urinary studies may all require sedation or general anaesthesia for the child's comfort and safety, particularly if the procedures are protracted and the children are young and frightened.

Radio-isotope scanning

Anaesthesia is very occasionally given to children undergoing radio-isotope scanning. The special problems encountered relate to the condition of the child and the room in which the scan is performed. The room is often small, with no piped gases or wall suction, and the staff are unused to anaesthetized patients. Monitoring and all anaesthetic apparatus will have to be brought into the room.

Magnetic resonance imaging (MRI)

MRI is a non-invasive investigation during which the patient must remain motionless for, usually, three or four periods of 10 min at a time, so the whole procedure may take between 30 and 60 min. The magnetic field, or bore surrounding the patient is long, noisy, and claustrophobic, and consequently small children usually require sedation (only partially satisfactory) or general anaesthesia to obtain acceptable images.[8]

General considerations

There is no risk of X-irradiation to the patient or the anaesthetist because the imaging does not involve X-rays. There is moreover, no known occupational hazard from frequent exposure to MRI. However, many of the general considerations listed earlier in this chapter apply equally to MRI (see earlier subsections on the environment, pre-investigation care, contrast media, and post-investigation care).

Specific considerations

Magnetic field   Imaging will be distorted by movement within the magnetic field and by the presence of ferromagnetic objects, which may also be drawn into the field, thus risking physical injury. The patient and all staff in or close to the scanner must leave outside the room certain wristwatches and coins, credit cards, keys, scissors, metal stethoscopes, laryngoscopes, and similar metal objects. Hospital trolleys must be removed before the imaging

11

Pain management in children

D. G. Hughes

It has been very difficult to improve the management of acute pain in children for a number of reasons. These include the inability to define and measure pain, the lack of appropriate equipment, psychological factors, and the great variation in analgesic requirements in the different age groups, neonates, infants, and children. However great strides have been made since Mather and Mackie reviewed the subject in 1983,[1] with greater emphasis on the use of regional analgesic techniques and the application of adult pain relief techniques to children (epidurals, patient-controlled analgesia), together with the development of appropriate techniques for studying pain in children.

It is difficult to measure pain directly and of the techniques used (subjective self-reporting scoring tests, plasma cortisol levels, plasma catecholamines, respiratory function tests) the linear analogue pain score (LAPS) is probably the most useful in adults. However, it requires patient understanding and cooperation. It has been modified for use in children by the addition of pictures (see Fig. 11.1) and Maunuksela *et al.*[2] found that as long as a face self-reporting scale is understood by a child pre-operatively it can be used as a measure of pain post-operatively (usually 4 years and over). They compared this scale with behavioural assessment of pain carried out by specially trained observers scoring pain on a scale from 0 (no pain) to 9 (worst possible pain) and found a highly significant correlation between behavioural assessment and self-reporting scales. However, the child must be able to understand the visual analogue scale and it cannot be used in children under 4 years of age or in infants and neonates. Other authors have used behavioural observation methods which do not rely upon the ability of the child to comprehend or communicate, that is,

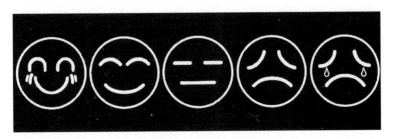

Fig. 11.1 Faces self-reporting scale.

they are independent of verbal skills. Many different systems are now available, mainly for use in research, but they may have an application in an acute pain service programme. They can be completed by the nursing staff, together with routine monitoring that is now carried out. This may be useful for severe pain but not so useful for mild to moderate pain.

POST-OPERATIVE PAIN RELIEF IN INFANTS AND CHILDREN

The rational use of analgesics in children relies on an individual approach to each child to allow for variability in pain, depending upon the type of surgery, the age of the child (differing pharmacokinetics, pharmacodynamics), and the availability of skilled nursing staff, perhaps in a high dependency unit if complicated techniques are to be used in small infants.

The use of opioids (see also Chapter 2)

Despite continuing research for new drugs, the opioids are still the most commonly used centrally acting analgesics during surgery and in the post-operative period. Their use as premedicant drugs has declined in recent years, with greater emphasis on the use of benzodiazepines to minimize anxiety pre-operatively. These opioids may be full or partial μ, κ, or δ receptor agonists, although experience in the use of agonist-antagonist drugs for children is limited. Morphine is popular and remains the standard drug against which other drugs are compared.

Morphine

This drug has been used as the standard analgesic drug for children using intermittent intramuscular injections but this often results in unsatisfactory analgesia due to the peaks and troughs in blood levels. However, children and nursing staff dislike injections ('*needles*') and, with greater understanding of the pharmacokinetics of morphine in children, continuous intravenous infusions are now employed. These infusions have been regularly used without respiratory complications and with a lower incidence of side-effects such as nausea and vomiting. Caution must be observed in infants, and guidelines should be given to both medical and nursing staff. Ideally the infusion should be run through a separate intravenous cannula and the dose should be titrated against the response of the child, using some form of pain scale, visual analogue, or objective pain score. The rate of the infusion should be set between 10 and 40 μg kg^{-1} h^{-1}, starting with a low dose and increasing the dose as required. A bolus dose of 100 μg kg^{-1} would need to be given initially if an appropriate dose of analgesic had not been given intra-operatively, or if the infusion was being used in the intensive care unit for sedation and analgesia. In a well-organized pain relief programme it should not be necessary to use top-up doses of morphine. The infusion should be run through a volumetric syringe pump whose accuracy should be regularly checked. These infusions must be used cautiously in any child with respiratory disease or obstruction of the upper respiratory tract, for example by large tonsils, or in mentally retarded children.

Dose: 0.5 mg kg^{-1}; make up to 50 ml with 5 per cent glucose or 0.9% saline. 1 ml h^{-1} = 10 μg kg^{-1} h^{-1}.

An opioid infusion (e.g. morphine) can provide good analgesia but may be associated with the following problems:

- OVER SEDATION AND VENTILATORY DEPRESSION. Marked ventilatory depression will only occur in a patient who is very sedated. If the patient is somnolent and difficult to arouse stop the infusion.

- FAILED ANALGESIA. This may be due to pump failure, loss of IV access or giving insufficient opioid drug. The syringe pump, the syringe, the extension line, and the IV cannula should be inspected.

Subcutaneous cannula for opioid administration
Intramuscular or repeated subcutaneous injections should be avoided in children. If only one or two injections might be required and an IV infusion or patient-controlled analgesia (PCA) are not justified, many children can be well managed using a *subcutaneous cannula*. A small IV cannula is placed subcutaneously in the theatre, and secured with 'Mefix'. Good sites are the lateral aspect of the thigh or abdominal wall. Small volume intermittent injections can then be made almost painlessly. This method is suitable for 24 hours use.

Morphine elixir (Oramorph)
This is effective but large doses are required due to 'first pass' metabolism. Constipation is a problem.

Sustained-release morphine (MST)
Morphine can have a prolonged delivery using a drug matrix as in MST continus (Napp) which gives sustained plasma morphine levels. However, MST does have a slower onset of action and would be unsuitable for titrating against acute pain when rapid changes are required.

Pethidine

Pethidine can be given slowly in a bolus dose of 1–2 mg kg^{-1} intravenously but for routine use does not have any advantages over morphine. Its atropine-like properties may, however, be beneficial in asthmatic children.

Codeine

Codeine can be used in combination with paracetamol for treating mild pain, especially in day case surgery and where local analgesic blocks have been used. It can be given intramuscularly in a dose of 1 mg kg^{-1} or as an oral elixir but must never be given intravenously as profound hypotension may occur.

Fentanyl

Fentanyl is not used as often as morphine as a continuous infusion because it has more variable pharmacokinetics. Its much greater lipid solubility produces long-lasting effects after the infusion is turned off and recovery can be very prolonged compared with morphine. The infusion dose for post-operative pain relief in children is 2–4 μg kg^{-1}h^{-1} with a loading dose of 1–2 μg kg^{-1}. A higher dose, 4–8 μg kg^{-1} h^{-1} might be used for sedation in an intensive care environment.

Alfentanil

The drug is less lipid soluble than fentanyl and may be better for post-operative infusion in children. However, very little work has been carried out on the use of alfentanil as a continuous post-operative infusion.

Sufentanil

There is very little data available on the use of sufentanil in children. Davis et al.[3] have administered bolus doses of 15 μg kg^{-1} to children undergoing cardiac surgery. They found that this dose blocked any cardiovascular response to surgical incision and sternotomy and suggested that infants and children have higher clearances than adults, with shorter elimination half-lives.

Partial agonist opioids

Buprenorphine is a highly lipid-soluble drug with a long duration of action which has been shown to be effective in children. The parenteral preparation has a longer duration of action than morphine, up to 6 h. The main advantage of the sublingual preparations is the ability to avoid injections, which are always unpopular in children. Maunuksela et al.[4] used the sublingual preparation (5–7 mg kg^{-1}) with good effect for post-operative pain relief following orthopaedic surgery.[4]

Dose: 3–6 mg kg^{-1}.

Nalbuphine

Another partial agonist, nalbuphine, has been used in children for relief of pain following a variety of surgical procedures.[5] It has been found to be as good as morphine with a similar incidence of side-effects, nausea, and vomiting. It has the advantage that a 'ceiling' on respiratory depressant effect is reached, probably associated with a ceiling in analgesic action. It is only available in a parenteral form.

Dose: $0.15-0.3$ mg kg^{-1}.

Cyclo-oxygenase inhibitors

This group includes the non-steroidal anti-inflammatory drugs (NSAIDs) and drugs such as paracetamol. They have been shown to be as effective as the opioids in many types of mild to moderate pain, and (except for paracetamol) especially where any degree of tissue inflammation contributes to the pain. Diclofenac has been used to relieve pain following tonsillectomy either as a rectal suppository or intramuscularly intra-operatively.[6] Ibuprofen has been used for post-operative pain relief following dental extractions in children and has proved to be more effective than paracetamol or paracetamol and codeine. One of the main disadvantages of NSAIDs is the tendency to increase or prolong post-operative bleeding and to worsen bronchospasm. (The association between aspirin and Reye's syndrome restricts the use of this drug to children over the age of 12 years).

Patient-controlled analgesia

This technique has been used for a number of years in adult practice and since the introduction of reliable commercially available microprocessor-operated infusion syringe pumps suitable for PCA, a number of centres have been routinely using this technique in children aged 6–15 years. There are two ways of using the technique, either utilizing on-demand bolus doses or using demand doses with a background infusion. Rodgers *et al.*,[7] using morphine sulphate in adolescents, employed a technique without any background infusions relying on bolus doses alone. They suggest a loading dose of morphine of $50-100$ μg kg^{-1} followed by a bolus dose of $25-50$ μg kg^{-1}. The lockout interval (the time during which another dose cannot be given irrespective of the child pressing the demand device) was 10–15 min and the maximum 4 h limit was $100-200$ μg kg^{-1} of morphine sulphate. They found that the technique was happily accepted by the child, parents, and the nursing staff. Gaukroger *et al.*[8] have used PCA in smaller children with a background infusion of 16 μg kg^{-1} h^{-1} of morphine sulphate, preceded by an appropriate bolus dose. A bolus dose of 16 μg kg^{-1} was administered and the lockout interval was 5 mins.

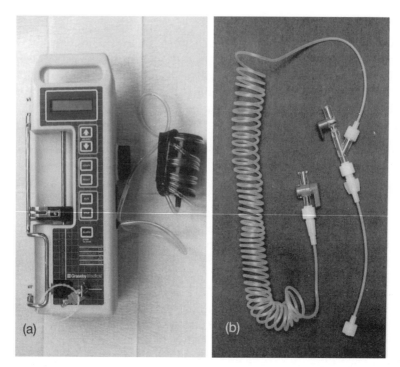

Fig. 11.3 (a) Patient-controlled analgesia syringe driver. (b) Delivery system showing one-way valve.

It is important to use an anti-reflux valve in the intravenous line if a dedicated line (cannula) is not used. Probably the main disadvantage of this technique is the price of the infusion pumps, together with the considerable education and training of the medical and nursing staff that is required. It is also a technique that cannot be used in a child who is unable to understand how to use the demand device and is therefore restricted to children over 6 years.

Patient selection

- Potential PCA patients will be identified prior to surgery. The post-operative management should be discussed with the child, parents, and the nurses looking after the child.

- Children six years and older and who are able to understand the PCA instructions and can push the PCA button.

- Children undergoing surgical procedures, when a child is expected to remain hospitalized longer than 24 hours and will require IV opioid analgesia. Acute pain episodes during a medical admission (e.g. sickle cell disease). Acute pain during treatment (e.g. mucositis with bone marrow transplants). Chronic pain management.

Patient assessment

- Assess if the child is willing and able to make the decision to manage their own pain and push the button.
- Determine the child's ability to discriminate painful stimuli.

PCA may be associated with the following problems:

- Sedation and ventilatory depression — The recognition of and response to over sedation is the same as for IV morphine infusions.
- Failed analgesia — This can result from the equipment failing to deliver the drug, or from the bolus dose being too small or the lockout time being too long.

The use of regional analgesic techniques

Regional analgesia was very popular in children in the early part of this century but as paediatric anaesthesia improved with the advent of muscle relaxants and halothane, so the popularity of local blocks declined. However, there has been an increased interest in regional analgesia in recent years with the introduction of the longer-acting local analgesic agent bupivacaine and the greater awareness of the need for good post-operative analgesia in children. These blocks can provide prolonged analgesia in the post-operative period by careful pre-operative planning and selection of the appropriate type of spinal, caudal, or epidural block or local analgesic technique that is used.

In adults it is easy to use regional analgesia as the sole technique for many operations, e.g. spinal for prostatectomy or total hip replacement. However, in children the regional analgesic technique is carried out once the child is asleep. Local analgesics reduce the requirement for opioid drugs and the use of high concentrations of volatile agents intra-operatively.

Pharmacokinetics of local analgesic agents in children

There are differences in the way in which local analgesic drugs are distributed and metabolized by the very young. In the infant, nerves are less myelinated than in adults and onset times tend to be shorter. Lower concentrations of drugs will result in a good block. Plasma protein concentrations are low at birth and do not reach adults levels until 6–12 months of age. Therefore because local analgesic drugs are bound to plasma proteins, albumen, and alpha acid glycoprotein (AAG), there is more active drug available in infants and especially in the neonate. There are also differences in metabolism, particularly the microsomal enzyme systems, and the neonate has a very limited capacity for metabolizing mepivacaine and bupivacaine. Infants eliminate local analgesic drugs at a faster rate than adults, possibly because of the relatively larger size of the liver in the child as a percentage of the total body weight with more sites for degradation of drugs. Eyres *et al.*,[9] using concentrations of 3 mg kg^{-1} bupivacaine for caudal blocks, found peak plasma concentrations in 1 year old of 1.4 μg ml^{-1} occurring about 10–15 mins after the block had been carried out as compared 30 mins in the adult, which is probably related to increased cardiac output.

It is important to be careful with doses of local analgesic drugs in infants (less than 1 year of age) but it would seem that older children are more tolerant of high doses (up to 4 mg kg^{-1} bupivacaine).

TECHNIQUES

Many blocks which are carried out in children can only be accomplished with the child anesthetized. It is important to explain to the child and to the parents about the type of block that is going to be used and the duration of analgesia that will be achieved. A good explanation of the side-effects (e.g. that a caudal block may produce heavy legs and loss of sensation), is also essential not only for the benefits of parents and child but also for the nursing staff. Out-patient surgery is increasing and the use of specific blocks and local infiltration will help to reduce unwanted side-effects such as nausea and vomiting associated with the use of opioid drugs in ambulatory patients.

Topical anaesthesia

This technique can be used for bronchoscopy and laryngoscopy in children in conjunction with general anaesthesia. The local anaesthetic is rapidly absorbed through the mucous membrane and 10 per cent lignocaine spray should be used (maximum 4–5 mg kg^{-1}).

Local analgesic (EMLA and amethocaine cream)

'EMLA' is a *E*utectic *M*ixture of *L*ocal *A*naesthetic agents, comprising prilocaine and lignocaine and can be used to prevent pain associated with venepuncture. It can be conveniently given at the same time as any sedative

Table 11.1 Dose of local analgesic agents for children

	Plain (mg kg^{-1})	Dose (mg kg^{-1}) with adrenalin 1/200 000
Bupivacaine	3	4
Lignocaine	6	9
Prilocaine	6	—

or other premedication but it needs to be in contact with the skin under an occlusive dressing for at least 60 mins and has a duration of action of approximately 3 h. Ideally the occlusive dressing should be removed 5 mins before the venepuncture to reduce the amount of vasoconstriction. Large repeated doses may cause methaemoglobinaemia. Amethocaine cream does not cause vasoconstriction and may be more suitable over less prominent veins.

Peripheral nerve blocks

There are certain blocks that are very popular in children, such as an ilio-inguinal block and penile block. However, all regional analgesia techniques used in adults can be successfully carried out in children as long as the practitioner is fully conversant with the techniques in an adult. Because the child is nearly always anaesthetized for a block it is preferable that a peripheral nerve stimulator is used to locate the nerve to avoid damage. Ideally short bevelled blunt needles should be used. These regional analgesic techniques can be found in many textbooks on the subject and the reader is referred to appropriate texts for further information.[10,11] In this section only blocks commonly used in children will be discussed.

Penile block

Circumcision and minor hypospadias surgery are common procedures carried out in small children. Dorsal nerve block of the penis can provide good postoperative pain relief for these procedures for up to 12 h.[12] For major hypospadias surgery, infiltrations at the base of the penis may interfere with the surgical technique and a caudal block would be more appropriate.

The anatomical distribution of the nerve has been well described by Brown *et al.*[13] The dorsal nerves are bilateral and run deep to Buck's fascia adjacent to the midline and supply the distal two-thirds of the penis (twigs of pudendal nerves S2–4).

In order to obtain a good block, most authors[12] recommend placing one or two injections deep to Buck's fascia on either side of the midline using 0.5 per cent plain bupivacaine in a dose of 0.2 ml kg^{-1}. It has been shown that occasionally there is a midline septum which prevents diffusion of local anaesthetic across the midline and hence the occasional need for bilateral blocks. *Adrenaline-containing solutions must never be used in the penis or other end organs.*

Ilio-inguinal and iliohypogastric nerve block

Orchidopexy and inguinal herniotomies are also common operations carried out in children and a block of both these nerves can provide good postoperative analgesia.

The nerves run deep to the external oblique aponeurosis and can be blocked by injection at a point medial and inferior to the anterior superior iliac spine using a 23 gauge short bevelled needle.

The doses used for this block vary considerably. Shandling and Steward[14] using 0.5 per cent bupivacaine recommended up to 2 mg kg^{-1} whereas Smith and Jones[15] recommend up to 2.5 mg per year of age of 0.5 per cent bupivacaine (a dose of 0.5 ml year of age^{-1}). Stow *et al.*[16] have looked at plasma bupivacaine concentrations using 0.5 per cent bupivacaine in a smaller dose than Shandling[14] of 1.25 mg kg^{-1} . They found venous plasma bupivacaine concentrations of less than 2 μg ml^{-1}, considerably lower than 4 μg ml^{-1} which is generally accepted as a safe maximum plasma concentration. It would seem that up to 2 mg kg^{-1} should be safe and the dose and concentrations of drug selected is an individual choice. It is a straightforward technique which provides good post-operative analgesia especially for day case surgery. The author uses 0.25 per cent bupivacaine in a total dose of 2 mg kg^{-1} giving 50 per cent initially followed by local infiltration of the wound by the surgeon at the end of the procedure with the remaining volume, remembering that often bilateral herniotomies are carried out.

It must be remembered that block of the ilio-inguinal and iliohypogastric nerves will produce only *cutaneous* analgesia. Unless the deeper structures are infiltrated under direct vision, additional intra-operative analgesia will be required.

For orchidopexy, the scrotal incision is usually in the distribution of the genital branch of the genitofemoral nerve and block of this nerve at the pubic tubercle or wound infiltration is required.

Intercostal blocks

These nerves can easily be blocked by the surgeon at the end of a thoracotomy. A dose of 1–2 ml of 0.25 per cent bupivacaine is infiltrated around each nerve under direct vision. Pneumothorax is a common complication if the block is not done under direct vision but a new approach to intercostal blocks has been recommended by Shelley and Park[17] in which the needle is kept parallel to the rib in the midaxillary line in an attempt to reduce the incidence of pneumothoraces.

Intrapleural block

Intrapleural instillation of local anaesthetic has been used in adults and children since 1986, but the ideal anaesthetic agent and dose still need evaluation. The catheter for continuous infusion is fixed in position posteriorly at the end of a thoracotomy. McIlvaine *et al.*[18] using 0.25 per cent bupivacaine with 1 200 000 adrenaline found significant drug accumulation at 24 h when running the infusion at 1.25–2.5 mg kg^{-1} h^{-1}. Queen *et al.*[19] using a single injection of 1 per cent prilocaine with adrenaline, achieved good post-operative analgesia in four children but further evaluation of continuous post-operative infusion needs to be carried out before it can be considered as a routine technique and it is condemned by some authors as unsafe.

Local infiltration

Local anaesthesia by wound infiltration at the end of surgery has proved to be very effective for pain relief in many procedures, including breast biopsy and herniorrhaphy in adults. Fell *et al.*[20] used 0.25 per cent bupivacaine in a dose of 0.5 ml kg^{-1} for day case herniotomy in children and found that it gave post-operative analgesia which was as good as a caudal block. This dose can be used for many operations including pyloromyotomy in infants.

Central blocks

Anatomy

The spinal cord and dural sac in neonates and infants terminates more caudally than in adults. In neonates the spinal cord can end at L3 with the dural sac at S2–4. By 12 months of age the spinal cord ends at L1. In premature and term neonates the intercristal line is at L5/S1 and at L5 in children. Unlike with adult techniques, the function of a central block in infants and children is to provide intra-operative and post-operative analgesia and is not usually the sole anaesthetic technique, although recently both spinal blocks and caudal blocks have been used as the sole technique in some premature neonates.

Spinal subarachnoid blocks

These blocks are not usually carried out in children because of the post-operative disadvantage of loss of motor power which many children do not like. Also it has no advantages over a caudal epidural block for long-term post-operative pain relief. However spinal anaesthesia has been used for premature neonates and those ex-premature neonates who have suffered the consequences of respiratory distress syndrome and may have required low-flow oxygen therapy for bronchopulmonary dysplasia. A spinal block is experienced hands may reduce the risks of general anaesthesia in this high-risk group of infants. The lumber puncture should be carried out below the L3 interspace to avoid damage to the spinal cord. This can easily be done with the infant in the lateral position, with the body but not the neck well flexed using a 24 or 25 gauge lumbar puncture needle. Once free flow of cerebrospinal fluid is seen, the appropriate dose of heavy or isobaric 0.5 per cent bupivacaine without adrenaline, is injected through a tuberculin syringe. Gallagher and Crean[21] administer 0.5 per cent bupivacaine using the formula 0.06 mg kg^{-1} + 0.1 ml to allow for needle dead space. Armitage[10] and other writers have used 0.25 per cent bupivacaine in 4 per cent glucose (i.e. heavy spinal solution) 0.13 ml kg^{-1} + needle dead space for infants less than 4 kg, and 0.07 ml kg^{-1} for larger children. It is important to immobilize the upper extremities to prevent undue wriggling and a dummy may be required to keep the child happy. It is still essential to monitor the infants with an apnoea monitor post-operatively whether a local or general anaesthetic is used.

The technique has been successfully used in older children with sedation or a distraction technique with no reported incidence of hypotension in children from 7 weeks to 13 years.

Caudal block

This is probably the most popular and useful block in children and can be used in all age groups to provide analgesia up to and including the umbilicus but is commonly used for procedures involving the sacral roots, circumcision, hypospadias surgery, and anal surgery. A single injection is usually used but more recently epidural catheters have been introduced through the sacrococcygeal membrane.

Anatomy

The anatomy differs from that of an adult in that the fusion of the sacral vertebrae is not complete until the age of 8 years. At the lower end of the sacrum is the sacral hiatus which is the unfused 5th sacral vertebral arch and is covered by the sacrococcygeal membrane.

The block is easy to perform with the child placed in the lateral decubitus position. A strict aseptic technique should be employed with either a no-touch technique or using gloves. A short 23 gauge needle attached to a syringe containing the appropriate volume of local anaesthetic or a styleted lumber puncture needle is inserted into the caudal space in the midline. Initially the angle of entry is 45° to the spine with the bevel of the needle facing the anaesthetist. Once the sacrococcygeal membrane is pierced the angle is flattened to about 15° and the needle is advanced 2–3 mm into the epidural space. Busoni and Sarti[22] have also used the cartilaginous 3rd and 4th sacral space in small children (less than 5 years, in whom the sacral vertebrae are not completely ossified).

Drugs and doses

Many different formulae have been used to determine the volume and concentrations of local anaesthetic required to obtain the level of analgesia for the surgery the child is undergoing. The regime of Armitage is probably the easiest to remember and is based on the weight of the child. He defined three areas to be blocked using different volumes of 0.25 per cent plain bupivacaine. A good lumbosacral sacral block (up to L1) results from 0.5 ml kg^{-1}. A dose of 1 ml kg^{-1} will block up to T10 (thoracolumbar) and 1.25 ml kg^{-1} will reach the mid-thoracic level (T6). Motor blockade can occur if 0.25 per cent bupivacaine is used but can be reduced by using 0.2 per cent or 0.166 per cent (see below). Other authors have used more complicated formulae and Schulte Steinberg and Rahlfs[23] found that there was a good correlation between age and dose requirement up to the age of 12 years. They state that a volume of approximately 0.1 ml of 1 per cent lignocaine or 0.25 per cent bupivacaine per segment per year of age was effective up to this age. Weight rather than age is probably a better guide to the volume of local anaesthetic required especially in very small infants.

The duration of action of a caudal block for surgery involving sacral roots using 0.25 per cent bupivacaine is probably less than 4 h and is much shorter for thoracolumbar and mid-thoracic blocks (about 2 to 3 h).

Eyres[9,24] has used concentrations of bupivacaine of 2 mg kg^{-1} and 3 mg kg^{-1}: with the low dose the venous plasma concentrations reached a maximum of 1 μg ml^{-1} and the highest concentration obtained with the higher dose was less than 1.4 μg ml^{-1} (the accepted maximum safe plasma level is 4 μg ml^{-1}).

Caudal morphine has recently been used for post-operative analgesia in children, with varying doses from 30 to 100 μg kg^{-1}.[25,26] The higher doses have given longer post-operative analgesia than when using 0.25 per cent bupivacaine alone.

A mixture of 0.125 per cent bupivacaine (0.75 ml kg^{-1}) and 50 μg kg^{-1} morphine has been shown to significantly improve post-operative pain relief following orchidopexy[27] although a higher concentration of bupivacaine 0.25 per cent with a similar concentration of morphine was needed for major hypospadias surgery.[28] Only one complication has been reported using morphine in the caudal epidural space,[29] that of Krane (delayed respiratory depression requiring naloxone in a 2 1/2 year old boy who received rather a high dose of 100 μg kg^{-1} of morphine), and until more work is carried out using these techniques these children should be monitored very closely in the post-operative period.

Complication

- Lack of success. Probably due to using the wrong volume of drug and inexperience in the technique.

- Intravenous injection. Can be avoided by repeated careful aspiration. If blood is seen in the syringe it is possible to reposition the needle and inject small volumes (0.5–1.0 ml) with careful aspiration between injections.

- Hypotension. This is rarely seen in children.

- Urinary retention. Again this is an uncommon problem unless the concentration of local anaesthetic is too high and a motor block results.

- Dural tap. The dural sac is lower in infants but this seems to be a rare complication in children. It may occur more commonly in newborns.

The duration of a caudal block can be prolonged by using a caudal catheter rather than a single dose technique. It is possible to advance a catheter to the lumbar or even thoracic level in small infants, using either an 18 or 19 gauge epidural pack, or a 23 gauge catheter passed into the epidural space through a 20 swg venous cannula.[30,31] There is a danger of infection, being so close to the anus, but this can be overcome by using a meticulous technique with sterile plastic adhesive dressings. Because the sacral vertebrae are not ossified in small children Busoni and Sarti[22] passed a catheter through the S2/3 space. The doses used for caudal lumbar catheters positioned at the L2 level are based on a modified formula of Takasaki *et al.*[31] (ml segments^{-1} = 0.0056 × body weight (kg)). Post-operatively an infusion of 0.25 per cent bupivacaine can be run at a rate of 0.1–0.2 ml kg^{-1} h^{-1} but probably not for more than 24 h because of the risk of infection from soiling. This technique and any form of epidural catheter must only be used in experienced hands.

Lumbar epidural block

As with spinal blocks this is not usually carried out as the sole anaesthetic technique in small children. It is technically more difficult than using the caudal approach but does have a place if prolonged post-operative analgesia is required.

A formula for estimating the distance from the skin to the lumbar epidural space in infants and children was suggested by Uemura and Yamashita.[33]

$$\text{Distance} = (\text{weight} + 10) \times 0.8$$

(weight in kilos; distance in mm)

The equipment is now available and Portex produce a 19 gauge Tuohy needle with a 23 gauge catheter. Epidural bupivacaine (0.5 ml kg^{-1} with 1 200 000 adrenaline) has been used by Dalens[34] with and without the addition of preservative-free morphine (50 μg kg^{-1}). This technique had an 8 per cent incidence of dural puncture which seems unacceptably high. The side-effects included itching, nausea, and vomiting, and urinary retention in those children who had morphine. However, the duration of analgesia was much longer (17–20 h compared to 3.75 to 4.5 h).

The catheters should be placed at the upper end of the higher dermatome of the surgical field in order to provide good post-operative analgesia using a continuous infusion. A test dose is normally used to exclude an intravascular or subarachnoid injection. However, in anaesthetized children it is probably not possible to detect an intravascular injection reliably, even by using local anaesthetic solution containing 1 : 20 000 adrenaline. The bolus dose used is 0.5–0.75 ml kg^{-1} of 0.25 per cent bupivacaine with half this dose as a top up. For continuous infusion post-operatively a dose of 0.1 ml kg^{-1} h^{-1} of 0.166 per cent bupivacaine can be used (20 ml 0.5 per cent bupivacaine + 40 ml

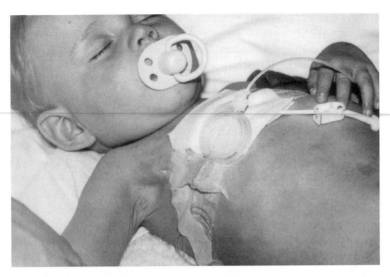

Fig. 11.2 Continuous post-operative epidural analgesia in a small child.

0.9 per cent saline) Diamorphine in a dose of 25 μg ml^{-1} can be added to 0.166% bupivacaine to potentiate the analgesia. Desparmet[35] has used an infusion of 0.25 per cent bupivacaine in a dose of 0.08 ml kg^{-1} h^{-1}. By using a low concentration of local anaesthetic, motor block is avoided and it will be adequate to block stress-mediated responses.

Hypotension again is not a problem in children but urinary retention may occur if there is any degree of motor block. Lumbar epidural catheters may be left in place for several days since the infection risk is small.

Thoracic epidural blocks

In order to achieve good analgesia for high abdominal surgery using the caudal route, large volumes of local anaesthetic would be required unless a catheter technique is employed. Some authors have used thoracic epidurals in children; they are obviously technically more difficult in small children but the same techniques and doses of local anaesthetic can be used. To obviate the problem of direct thoracic epidurals, some authors have used the caudal approach to the thoracolumbar region in infants and found it to be a safe technique.[30] These techniques can be very difficult and more work is required before they can be recommended for routine use.

Epidural infusion for pain relief

Epidural infusions can provide excellent analgesia but some unwanted effects may occur. These include hypotension, leg weakness, difficulty in micturition, and occasionally difficulty in breathing. These effects occur because the local anaesthetic blocks all types of nerve fibres, not just those responsible for pain.

Leg weakness — the patient may sit out in a chair but should be told not to attempt to walk. By the time the patients are ready to move/walk the epidural will most probably have been removed.

Difficulty in micturition — a bedpan or urinary catheter should be used as required. The patient should not walk to the lavatory.

Hypotension — This is rare in young children but becomes more common with increasing age. The first response should be to exclude other causes of hypotension, in particular post-operative haemorrhage. Most cases will respond to a bolus of intravenous fluids. Nausea may be the first symptom of severe hypotension (do not give anti-emetics without first checking the blood pressure).

Over-sedation and ventilatory depression — Ventilatory depression never occurs in a patient who is awake and alert. Patients at risk of opioid-induced ventilatory depression are very sedated and difficult to arouse. It is for this reason that the sedation score should be recorded. Recording ventilatory rate is really only useful as a safeguard against ventilatory depression when the patient is felt to be experiencing normal sleep. Over-sedation tends to occur in patients who are given opioids by a combination of both epidural and other routes. For this reason, no patient with an epidural infusion containing opioids should receive any oral, IM, or IV opioids. If the patient is somnolent and difficult to arouse, stop the infusion. It is particularly important that other doctors discuss follow-up (post-operative) analgesia with the anaesthetic team to avoid this danger.

Failure to provide pain relief — This is usually due to the catheter no longer being in the epidural space or failure of the analgesic solution to reach one or more nerve roots. The dressings over the epidural should be inspected for fluid leaks. There may be a number of reasons why the epidural is not apparently working.

- *Problem*: The infusion is set at too low a rate.
  Treatment: Increase the rate of infusion to maximum of the range prescribed and consider a bolus top-up dose.
- *Problem*: The child may have a full bladder — this may cause distress and it may be thought that the epidural is not working
  Treatment: Check to see if the child has a full bladder. Bladder catheterization may be required.
- *Problem*: In some children following orthopaedic procedures muscle spasms may cause pain.
  Treatment: Set up a low-dose midazolam infusion if not already running (25–50 μg kg^{-1} h^{-1}).

- *Problem*: The catheter is not in the epidural space.
  Treatment: Check the site of the epidural catheter. It may be necessary to change to another technique — e.g. morphine infusion.

MONITORING THE CHILD

1. BP and pulse (and respiratory rate if opioid is being administered)

- The pulse rate and blood pressure should be recorded quarter hourly for the first hour, or while the child's condition is unstable.
- Half hourly for the next two hours.
- Hourly for the first twelve hours.
- Nursing judgement should be exercised regarding frequency of additional vital signs measurements. (e.g. 2–3 hourly)

2. Sedation level

- Numbers on scale 0–3 (0 = awake and alert; 3 = somnolent, difficult to arouse) should be recorded with vital signs observations.
- REMEMBER – somnolence and increased drowsiness usually precedes respiratory depression. If the child is unrousable, switch off the pump and give oxygen. Titrated small doses of naloxone (1 μg kg^{-1} IV) should be given until the child is easily rousable and can answer questions.

> **BEWARE OF PRECIPITATING ACUTE PAIN AND STRESS BY OVER-ZEALOUS REVERSAL**

> *NALOXONE WILL ONLY BE EFFECTIVE IF THE PATIENT HAS RECEIVED AN OPIOID. RESPIRATORY DIFFICULTIES DUE TO A HIGH LEVEL LOCAL ANAESTHETIC BLOCK MUST BE TREATED WITH OXYGEN AND ARTIFICIAL VENTILATION IF REQUIRED.*

3. Pain assessment

- The number scale 0–3 (0 = no pain; 1 = mild; 2 = moderate; 3 = severe pain) can be used to assess the quality of pain relief.
- Pain scores should also be recorded at time intervals as for vital signs above.

REFERENCES

1. Mather, L. and Mackie J. (1983). The incidence of postoperative pain in children. *Pain*, **15**, 271.
2. Maunuksela, E. L., Olkkola, K. T., and Korpela, R. (1987). Measurement of pain in children with self reporting and behavioural assessment. *Clinical Pharmacology and Therapeutics*, **42**, 137.
3. Davis, P. J., *et al.* (1987). Pharmacodynamics and pharmacokinetics of high dose sufentanil in infants and children undergoing cardiac surgery. *Anesthesia and Analgesia*, **66**, 203.
4. Maunuksela, E. L. Korpela, R., and Olkkola, K. T. (1988). Double-blind multiple dose comparison of buprenophine and morphine in postoperative pain in children. *British Journal of Anaesthesia*, **66**, 48.
5. Hughes, D. G. (1988). Nalbuphine for post operative pain relief in children. *Pain*, **9**, 52.
6. Walters, C. H. *et al.* (1988). Diclofenac sodium for post-tonsillectomy pain in children. *Anaesthesia*, **43**, 641.
7. Rodgers, B. M. *et al.* (1988). Patient controlled analgesia in pediatric surgery. *Journal of Pediatric Surgery*, **33**, 259.
8. Gaukroger, P. B., Tomkins, D. P., and Vander Walt, J. H. (1989). Patient controlled analgesia in children. *Anaesthesia and Intensive Care*, **17**, 264.
9. Eyres, R. L. *et al.* (1983). Plasma bupivacaine concentrations in children during caudal epidural analgesia. *Anaesthesia and Intensive Care*, **11**, 20.
10. Peutrell, J. M. and Mather, S. J. (1996). *Local anaesthesia for babies and children*. Oxford University Press.
11. Arthur, D. S. and McNichol, L. E. (1986). Local anaesthetic techniques in paediatric surgery *British Journal of Anesthesia*, **58**, 760.
12. White, J., Morrison, B., Richmond, P., Procter, A., and Carron, J. (1983). Postoperative analgesia for circumcision. *British Medical Journal*, **286**, 1934.
13. Brown, T. C. K., Weidner, N. J., and Bouwmester, J. (1989). Dorsal nerve of penis block — anatomical and radiological studies. *Intensive Care*, **17**, 34.
14. Shandling, B. and Steward, D. S. (1980). Regional analgesia for postoperative pain in pediatric outpatient surgery. *Journal of Pediatric Surgery*. **15**, 477.
15. Smith, S. A. C. and Jones, S. E. F. (1982). Analgesia after herniotomy in a paediatric day unit. *British Medical Journal*, **285**, 1466.
16. Stow, P. J., Scott, A., Phillips, A., and White, J. B. (1988). Plasma bupivacaine concentrations during caudal analgesia and ilioinguinal-iliohypogastric nerve block in children. *Anaesthesia*, **43**, 650.
17. Shelly, M. P. and Park, G. R. (1987). Intercostal nerve blockade for children. *Anaesthesia*, **42**, 541.
18. McIlvaine, W. B., Knox, R. F., Fennessey, P. V., and Goldstein, M. (1988). Continuous infusion of bupivacaine via intrapleural catheter for analgesia after thoracotomy in children *Anesthesiology*, **69**, 261.

19. Queen, J. S., Kahana, M. D., Difazio, C. A., Noble, H. A., and Rodgers, B. M. (1989). An evaluation of interpleural analgesia with etidocaine in children. *Anesthesia and Analgesia*, **68**, 51.
20. Fell, D., Denington, M. C., Taylor, E., and Wandless, J. G. (1988). Paediatric postoperative analgesia. A comparison between caudal block and wound infiltration of local anaesthetic. *Anaesthesia*, **43**, 107.
21. Gallagher, T. M. and Crean, P. M. (1989). Spinal anaesthesia in infants born prematurely. *Anaesthesia*, **44**, 434.
22. Busoni, P. and Sarti, A. (1987). A sacral intervertebral epidural block. *Anesthesiology*, **67**, 993.
23. Schulte Steinberg, O. and Rahlfs, V. W. (1977). Spread of extradural analgesia following caudal injection in children. *British Journal of Anaesthesia*, **49**. 1027.
24. Eyres, R. L., Kidd, J., Oppenheim, R. C., and Brown, T. C. K. (1978). Local anaesthetic plasma levels in children. *Anaesthesia and Intensive Care*, **6**, 243.
25. Jensen, B. H. (1981). Caudal block for post operative pain relief in children after genital operations. A comparison between bupivacaine and morphine. *Acta Anaesthesiologica Scandinavica*, **25**, 373.
26. Krane, F. J. *et al.* (1987). Caudal morphine for postoperative analgesia in children: a comparison with caudal bupivacaine and intravenous morphine. *Anaesthesia and Analgesia*, **66**, 647.
27. Wolf, A. R. *et al.* (1990). Postoperative analgesia after paediatric orchidopexy. The evaluation of a bupivacaine/morphine mixture. *British Journal of Anaesthesia*, **64**, 430.
28. Wolf, A. R. *et al.* (1989). Combined bupivacaine/morphine caudals; duration of analgesia and plasma morphine concentration. *Anesthesiology*, **70**, A1015.
29. Krane, E. J. (1988). Delayed respiratory depression in a child after caudal epidural morphine. *Anesthesia and Analgesia*, **67**, 79.
30. Boösenberg, A. T., Bland, B. A., Schulte-Steinberg, O., and Downing, J. W. (1988). Thoracic epidural anaesthesia via the caudal route in infants. *Anesthesiology*, **69**, 265.
31. Peutrell, J. M. and Hughes, D. G. (1994). Combined spinal and epidural anaesthesia for inguinal hemia repair in babies. *Paediatric Anaesthesia*, **4**, 221.
32. Takasaki M. *et al.* (1977). Dosage for caudal anaesthesia in infants and children. *Anesthesiology*, **47**, 527.
33. Uemura, A. and Yamashita, M. (1992). Formula for determining the distance from the skin to the lumbar epidural space in infants and children. *Paediatric Anaesthesia*, **2**, 305.
34. Dalens, B., Tanguy, A., and Harberer, J. P. (1986), Lumbar epidural anaesthesia for operative and postoperative pain relief in infants and young children. *Anesthesia and Analgesia*, **65**, 1069.
35. Desparmet, J. *et al.* (1987). Continuous epidural infusion of bupivacaine for postoperative pain relief in children. *Anesthesiology*, **67**, 108.

FURTHER READING

Armitage, E. N. (1979). Caudal block in children. *Anaesthesia*, **34**, 396.
Bradman, L. M. *et al.* (1990). Parent-assisted PCA for postoperative pain control in young children. *Anesthesia and Analgesia*, **70**, (1990). Suppl. 34.

Cox, R. G. and Goresky, G. V. (1990). Life-threatening apnea following spinal anaesthesia in former premature infants. *Anesthesiology*, **73**, 345.

Lawrie, S. C. *et al.* (1990). Patient controlled analgesia in children. *Anaesthesia*, **45**, 1074.

Lloyd-Thomas, A. R. (1990). Pain management in paediatric patients. *British Journal of Anaesthesia*, **64**, 85.

Weight, T. E. *et al.* (1990). Complications during spinal anaesthesia in infants — high spinal blockade. *Anesthesiology*, **73**, 1290.

12

Acute airway problems

S. J. Mather

Most of the conditions anaesthetists are asked to be involved with urgently are upper airway difficulties (Table 12.1), most commonly laryngotracheo-bronchitis (croup), more rarely acute epiglottitis, or mechanical obstruction of the airway. Inhalation of a foreign body must always be considered in small children (under 4).

SIGNS OF AIRWAY OBSTRUCTION

Stridor

Stridor is the musical or squeaky sound produced when air traverses the partially obstructed upper airway. It may be inspiratory or expiratory. Often

Table 12.1   Acute airway problems

Congenital	Acquired
Choanal atresia	Loss of airway control
Large tongue (e.g. Beckwith syndrome)	Acute epiglottitis
	Laryngotracheobronchitis
Craniofacial anomalies (e.g.	Inhaled foreign body
Pierre Robin syndrome)	Peritonsillar abscess
Subglottic stenosis	Diphtheria (rare)
Laryngo- and tracheomalacia	Ludwig's angina (rare)
Laryngeal and tracheal stenosis	Trauma (including intubation)
Laryngeal web	Chemical and thermal injury
Vascular ring or sling	Subglottic stenosis
Nerve palsies and neuromuscular	Nerve palsies
disorders	Tumours
Tumours (e.g. haemangiomata, cystic	Allergies — angioneurotic oedema
hygroma)	
	Other medical conditions:
	Juvenile rheumatoid
	Acute asthma
	Pneumonia with copious secretions
	Bronchiolitis

both inspiratory and expiratory stridor are present. Stridor in inspiration is due to laryngeal obstruction, whereas expiratory stridor largely originates below the larynx.

Intercostal recession

Intercostal and subcostal recession and 'see-sawing' of the abdomen indicate obstruction. Intercostal recession is easily seen in babies due to the greater elasticity of their chest walls. The relatively large negative pressures generated in an attempt to overcome the obstruction results in indrawing of the chest wall structures and abdomen. The paradoxical see-saw motion of the abdomen during the inspiratory effort is characteristic.

Assessment

Time should be devoted to obtaining as complete a history as possible. The differential diagnosis is wide and previous similar incidents may point one in the right direction, although one must be alert to the possibility that a different cause may be responsible on this occasion. This is especially true of the child with an inhaled foreign body which may mimic almost every other cause of acute upper airway obstruction, particularly croup.

Particular difficulty exists in the case of a child with severe acute epiglottitis. Such a child may suffer fatal hypoxia if handled to examine his chest or throat or to put up a drip. If this condition is suspected, the child must not be handled other than to administer a general anaesthetic (see below).

Less severely ill children should have their chest examined, the temperature taken, and, if appropriate, a white cell count, sedimentation rate, and chest radiograph obtained. Wheezing children should not be subjected to respiratory function tests when they are in respiratory distress. These should be reserved for evaluation after treatment.

Occasionally a child with respiratory distress is referred from a district hospital without full facilities for its care. In this instance a retrieval team from the regional centre should undertake to collect the child. The team must include an anaesthetist experienced enough to deal with acute upper airway obstruction and a possible difficult intubation. In some cases it may be preferable for that anaesthetist to intubate the child under general anaesthesia at the referring hospital to enable a safe transfer to be made.

SPECIFIC CONDITIONS

Only those conditions which commonly cause problems for the anaesthetist will be discussed here. For discussion of the other conditions mentioned in Table 12.1 the reader is referred to standard texts.

The anaesthetic department is usually asked to be involved with the management of the child by the paediatricians or accident and emergency staff when hypoxia has occurred or ventilatory failure is anticipated. Mostly this will be due to acquired conditions but occasionally congenital problems (e.g. cysts, tumours, or subglottic stenosis) present acutely.

ACUTE EPIGLOTTITIS

This condition is rather rare compared with croup which is the main differential diagnosis. It is becoming even rarer now that immunization is available. It is caused by infection with *Haemophilus influenzae* type B and mostly occurs in children under 5 years of age. A vaccine active against *Haemophilus influenzae* type B (HIB vaccine) is now offered as part of the routine immunization programme in the UK. In acute epiglottitis there is rapidly developing oedema of the epiglottis and aryepiglottic folds. The oedema can virtually close the airway to a pinhole within a few hours. The child is typically very toxic and exhausted, with a high fever, and cannot swallow his saliva, which drools from the mouth. There is intense sore throat, but the child cannot drink or speak.

On no account must the pharynx be examined or the child sent for X-ray examination.

Fatalities have occurred when a tongue depressor or laryngoscope have been used to get a better view of the pharynx. Soft tissue lateral neck radiographs have been advocated but are of little help and may put the child's life at risk. Nothing should be done to the child prior to general anaesthesia. No attempt should be made to put up a drip or to make the child answer questions.

Anaesthetic management

Gentle and unhurried inhalational induction of anaesthesia with 100 per cent oxygen and halothane is preferred, maintaining spontaneous ventilation. This should be the first therapeutic manoeuvre. Acute epiglottitis is a positive indication for halothane. No other agent should be used unless there is an absolute contraindication (e.g. proven malignant hyperpyrexia susceptibility).

On laryngoscopy the typical appearance of the inflamed epiglottis is of a red cherry-shaped structure with a median groove. In severe cases it may only be possible to detect the laryngeal inlet by the appearance of small bubbles beneath the grossly swollen epiglottis.

Intubation may be extremely difficult, even in expert hands, and an endotracheal tube several sizes smaller in diameter than expected for the child's age and weight may be required. Pre-cut tubes may be too short; it is im-

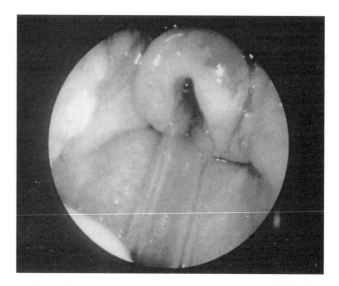

Fig. 12.1 Acute epiglottitis with endotracheal tube *in situ*.
(Photo: B. Smalhout.)

portant to make sure that a tube of sufficient length for the child is used. Expected sizes for tube lengths can be obtained from Oakley's chart (see Fig. 14.3).

Only very rarely is tracheostomy required but the means to perform it must be immediately to hand. Some authorities advocate insufflation with oxygen through a cricothyroid catheter (needle cricothyrotomy). It is vital to realize that gas must then have a route of escape through the larynx. *A second catheter does not allow the gas to escape adequately*. Tidal ventilation is not possible through small catheters. Such a manoeuvre can, at best, only provide the few minutes necessary to perform a tracheostomy sufficient to pass a small endotracheal tube.

Following nasal intubation, the child should be nursed in an intensive care unit breathing spontaneously on continuous positive airway pressure (CPAP) of about 5 cmH$_2$O. A small amount of added oxygen may be necessary. Occasionally these patients require mechanical ventilation for pulmonary complications such as collapse and consolidation.

Drug therapy consists of treatment with intravenous ampicillin, chloramphenicol, or cefuroxime. Resistance to ampicillin or chloramphenicol is less common in the UK than in some other countries.[1,2] Continuous intravenous sedation with benzodiazepines (e.g. midazolam) and perhaps low-dose opioids is required for 24–48 h. As the oedema subsides, evidenced by the increased leak around the tube, the fever settles and the child is able to swallow.

Some anaesthetists then perform a further laryngoscopy under anaesthesia to confirm resolution of the swelling. Others do not, believing that a good leak around the tube on applying 20 cmH$_2$O positive pressure to the circuit is sufficient evidence to perform extubation. This is accomplished in most cases within 48–72 h. Steroids should not be given in an attempt to hasten resolution of the oedema. Stridor may occur following extubation and should be treated with nebulized adrenaline (3–5 ml of 1 mg ml^{-1} solution, i.e. 1 in 1000 at any age).

Pulmonary oedema may rarely occur in association with acute epiglottitis.[1]

CROUP (LARYNGOTRACHEOBRONCHITIS)

This condition affects all the conducting airways. It is usually viral in origin, commonly due to influenza or para-influenza viruses. Respiratory syncitial virus is less often the cause. Croup mostly affects the 6 month to 2 years age group but older children are also susceptible. Most cases are seen in the winter months. Although usually viral, 'bacterial croup' is being increasingly seen with staphylococci, *Haemophilus influenzae,* and streptococci isolated from the tracheal aspirate. Secondary bacterial infection is very common following mucosal damage by the virus. The onset and progression of croup are slower than in acute epiglottitis and the illness may last 10–14 days. The child usually has a 'cold' with classical upper respiratory signs, progressing to a barking cough (croup).

Most cases can be treated at home and even of those admitted to hospital the vast majority (97 per cent) do not require airway support. Those which do are exhausted due to respiratory obstruction. Intravenous fluids are required to prevent dehydration but excessive fluid load should be avoided because water retention may occur.[3]

Nebulized adrenaline in the racemic form is widely used in North America for the treatment of croup and may help to avoid intubation. This preparation is not available in the UK but Remington and Meakin recommend the use of L-adrenaline (1 mg ml^{-1}) in a nebulized dose of 5 ml at any age, regardless of weight.[4] The effect of nebulized adrenaline is short, only about 2 h, so frequent administration may be required.[5]

Adrenaline is thought to work in this condition by alpha-adrenergic effects on the inflamed subglottic mucosa, producing vasoconstriction and thus reducing oedema.[4] A 30 per cent reduction in airway resistance has been reported.[6] This method of treatment is now considered safe and effective. There are usually few, if any, cardiovascular adverse effects beyond mild tachycardia but ECG monitoring is mandatory to detect dysrhythmia.

Steroids are not routinely employed, as there is no convincing evidence of their efficacy in croup, but a single dose of dexamethasone (0.5 mg kg^{-1}) may be given 6–12 h prior to extubation in an attempt to reduce post-extubation oedema, especially in those with a previous history of croup who are thought to have a tendency to increased bronchial reactivity.

Inhalation of steam or mist is no longer considered particularly helpful so long as the inspired gas is adequately humidified.

A clinical scoring system has been devised by Downes *et al.*[7] to assist in the assessment of severity of croup. (see Table 12.2). A croup score of 7 or more, especially in the presence of low oxygen saturation on pulse oximetry, which persists despite conservative treatment, suggests that endotracheal intubation is required. *Blood gas measurements may distress the child and worsen hypoxia, thus they should be avoided prior to anaesthesia.*

Intubation under general anaesthesia is required if the child is becoming exhausted. Many children can subsequently be managed with mild sedation until they can tolerate the tracheal tube, which may have to remain *in situ* for 2 weeks. A proportion will require ventilation for lower respiratory tract involvement, pneumonia, or simply because they are exhausted. Rapid weaning through intermittent mandatory ventilation (IMV) to CPAP is usually possible. Children with croup should be anaesthetized in the same way as those with acute epiglottitis, that is with oxygen and halothane. *Once the larynx has been visualized,* suxamethonium may be given if required. The tube size will be dictated by the size of the upper airway and must be decided empirically.

Extubation following croup

When the child is afebrile with a minimum of secretions, extubation can be considered if there is a good leak around the tube. If stridor persists it is wise to examine the airway under anaesthesia following croup since granulomata may form, resulting in the necessity for their endscopic removal. Humidified, oxygen-enriched air should be supplied for 24 h following extubation.

Table 12.2   Clinical scoring system for assessment of croup

Score	0	1	2
Inspiratory breath sounds	Normal	Harsh, with rhonchi	Delayed
Stridor	None	Inspiratory	Inspiratory and expiratory
Cough	None	Hoarse cry	Barking cough
Nasal flaring, suprasternal retraction, and intercostal recession	None	Flaring with retraction	Flaring, suprasternal, subcostal, and intercostal recession
Cyanosis	None	Cyanosed in air	Cyanosed in 40 per cent O_2
Sensorium	No change	Restless	Obtunded

to peripheral vasoconstriction and an increased heart rate.[3] Poor heating and cramped conditions are also problematical and often only one medical attendant can be carried. Monitoring equipment may be limited if the flight crew feel that the equipment might emit electromagnetic radiation that could interfere with navigational equipment. In the UK the road ambulance is the usual form of transport and although slower than helicopters it does have the advantage of a single transfer.

It has become evident that a transport team from the receiving centre is best able to organize the resuscitation of small infants. However, as the experience and skills of the peripheral Special Care Baby Units (SCBU) has improved, many units are able to provide their own transport teams. The facilities and care provided should be up to the same standard that would be expected in an Intensive Care environment.

The transport facilities, often referred to as secondary referrals, are required to transfer neonates, infants, and children for many reasons:

- Transfer from a District General Hospital to a specialized unit: SCBU, PICU, ICU, renal, burns, or neurosurgical unit where greater expertise is available.
- Inter-hospital/district transfer of children for further investigations not located on site because they are expensive or expertise is not available, e.g. renal dialysis, CT scan, MRI scan.
- Within-hospital transfer of children for surgery or for investigations (radiology). Neonates should arrive in the operating theatre ready for surgery in the optimum condition, i.e. warm, well-hydrated.
- Transfer of children from a specialized unit to the referring hospital for further, less-specialized care.
- Paediatric expertise should also be available for major disasters both for resuscitation, technical skills, and perhaps transport.

WHY IS A TRANSPORT TEAM REQUIRED?

- Preparation, including stabilization and perhaps resuscitation, of the child before embarking on a difficult journey. This may take a few hours and must be understood by the ambulance personnel.
- By utilizing a trolley and incubator unit together, it is possible to reduce the number of transfers of the child from trolley to trolley and so reduce the risk of accidental extubation. This makes the journey much easier and safer.
- Temperature control is vital in small neonates, and modern incubators have considerably improved the ability to keep an adequate thermoneutral environment.

- Airway management. The airway must be carefully assessed prior to transfer and if there are any doubts it is better to intubate the child and ventilate during the journey.

- Infusion of fluids, drugs, and monitoring can now easily be carried out using battery-powered syringe pumps.

- Monitoring required for the journey may include electrocardiogram, respiratory rate, temperature, transcutaneous PO_2, oxygen saturation, and perhaps blood pressure.

The provision of mobile intensive care for the neonate is now a well-recognized service. But it is only recently that physicians have recognized the need for improved transfer of infants and older children. This has been highlighted in recommendations from a working party set up by the British Paediatric Association on Paediatric Intensive Care. They recommended that PICUs should be adequately staffed to allow them to provide a 'fetch-and-carry' service. Complex cases should normally be discussed with the regional PICU staff and transfer then considered.

Even in 1981, Gentleman and Jennet demonstrated that simple measures were being ignored in the transfer of comatose head-injured children between hospitals.[4] The Royal Melbourne Children's Hospital set up their Paediatric Emergency Transport system in 1979, and developed the service rapidly because of the close links between the transport team and the St John's Ambulance Service and the need to transfer children for long distances safely.[5]

The medical team is probably the most important part of the system and they must be well-trained in resuscitation and management of sick infants, although much of the success of the retrieval teams is due to improved technology. The team should consist of a doctor and nurse and it often takes a few hours to stabilize a sick child; for example, a child with cyanotic heart disease may require a prostaglandin infusion, new intravenous lines may need to be set up, and simple measures like passing a nasogastric tube may be necessary. The child must not be moved into the ambulance until the team are satisfied that it is in the optimum condition for the journey. This may also include elective intubation if the child is very sick, in order to secure the airway and to prevent further hypoxia in a very sick infant. The experience from Melbourne has shown that 50 per cent of their children needed to be re-intubated and they selected the nasal route for children which they felt was safer, with less risk of inadvertent extubation and endobronchial intubation.

TRANSPORT SYSTEMS

- Transport systems consist of a number of important parts:
  transport incubator/trolley;

- ventilation;
- monitoring equipment;
- drugs — equipment.

Incubators

These have improved considerably in the last 5 years, with better temperature control and less heat loss by using double-skinned plastic canopies. It is important to have easy access to the infant and good visibility during transfer. A bubble plastic shield can be used to cover the infant to prevent further heat loss. It must be remembered that if an infant is cold, aluminized 'space' blankets do not transmit heat and cannot be used in an incubator to warm an infant, but merely to reduce heat loss.

Different incubators have different techniques for maintaining the incubator temperature which mainly rely on a source of power, such as a battery on the trolley unit with leads that can connect to the power supply of the ambulance. The unit has to be able to function on its own without electricity and with a limited oxygen supply. Air is necessary for neonates and can be provided by means of a lightweight portable compressor powered by a battery.

Ventilators

Many of the old incubators had a built in Vickers neovent ventilator which is not really adequate for present day ventilation. Newer ventilators, such as the Sechrist and Dräger Babylog, can be used with a mixer to permit inspired oxygen to be controlled between 21 and 100 per cent. Continuous positive airway pressure (CPAP), intermittent mandatory ventilation (IMV), and positive end expiratory pressure (PEEP) are also possible with these newer ventilators. For older children the Dräger Oxylog can be used; these are time-cycled ventilators, the respiratory frequency of which can be set by a simple dial. In the event of a ventilator failure, a back up T-piece system or self-inflating bag can be used and must always be carried in the emergency box.

Monitoring and infusion equipment

Again, great strides have been made in the design of portable monitoring equipment, many of which are now battery-powered (the battery life must be frequently checked). The following should be monitored:

- heart rate;
- respiratory rate;
- transcutaneous oxygen — neonates;
- oxygen saturation;

- temperature of incubator and infant;
- inspired oxygen;
- blood pressure — this is not a very easy task.

In our system, a DC to AC converter is carried with the transport system enabling the use of an ambulance or aircraft DC electrical supply. A monitor combining a number of parameters reduces the bulk of the equipment. The incubator is carried on a trolley which replaces the existing trolley in an ambulance and can be locked safely in place. The unit has the facility to be connected to the ambulance power and oxygen supplies, and the ambulance should be kept at 24 °C if possible.

In order to infuse drugs and fluids, battery-operated syringe pumps are employed and volumetric infusions can be used for long periods without mains power.

The system used in our hospital[6] has been modified to incorporate facilities for all age groups, neonates, infants, and children. It is based on a Dräger 5300 incubator. The basic trolley has been modified to accept either an incubator or a trolley mattress. All the monitoring equipment, syringe pumps, and ventilator are attached to the trolley.

ORGANIZATION

Communications

Referral calls are accepted from hospitals giving either a reason for referral or asking for advice. Special problems need to be discussed and arrangements can be made by the PICU coordinating doctor to arrange transfer of the team and equipment to the referring hospital and then to the appropriate specialized unit.[7]

Preparation

Notify ambulance control to collect the medical team and ensure that the appropriate transport trolley has been thoroughly checked.

Request police escort — depending upon urgency and time of day in large cities.

Road ambulance is the standard transport — occasionally a helicopter may be used.

Intensive Care staff need to prepare the bed space for the child, e.g. is a ventilator needed?; the number of infusion pumps required.

Flying squad case. This should contain:

- emergency drugs and a selection of drugs used routinely, e.g. antibiotics, muscle relaxants;

- airway management equipment and chest drainage equipment (including Heimlich valves) for all age groups;
- intravenous therapy equipment, including facility for umbilical artery cannulation and central venous cannulation;
- paediatric resuscitation equipment.

Audit — It is important to keep a good record of transfers, including the time of day and the length of time away. It is also important to keep a record of important clinical details such as temperature, drug infusions, and whether ventilated or otherwise.

Standardization of equipment is important and the minilink 8.5/15 mm system saves unnecessary changing of endotracheal tubes.

REFERENCES

1. Hackel, A. (1975). A medical transport system for the neonate. *Anesthesiology*, **43**, 258.
2. Gilligan, A. *et al.* (1977). Retrieval of the critically ill in South Australia. A co-ordinated approach. *The Medical Journal of Australia*, **24/31**, 849.
3. Campbell, A. N., Lightstone, A. D., Smith, J. M., Kirpalani, H., and Perlman, M. (1984). Mechanical vibration and sound levels experienced in neonatal transport. *American Journal of Diseases of Children*, **138**, 967.
4. Gentleman, D. and Jennet, B. (1981). Hazards of interhospital transport of comatose head injuries, *Lancet*, **ii**, 853.
5. Owen, J. and Duncan, A. W. (1983). Towards safer transport of sick and injured children. *Anaesthesia and Intensive Care*, **11**, 113.
6. Hughes, D. G. and Mather, S. J. (1987). Paediatric transport revisited. *Today's Anaesthetist*, **7**, 108.
7. Dorman, T. (1994). Transport of the critically ill child. *Care of the Critically Ill*, **10**, (2), 80.

14

Paediatric life support

S. J. Mather

Definitive guidelines for paediatric resuscitation have been published.[1]

Even the experienced paediatric anaesthetist may find difficulty in resuscitating the collapsed and apnoeic baby. For the occasional paediatric anaesthetist in a general hospital, perhaps less used to paediatric needs, the situation may be terrifying.

It is essential to remember that the principles of resuscitation remain the same. Attention to ABC (airway, breathing, and circulation) using simple measures may be effective in themselves. It is rarely necessary to rush to intubate the child, better to ventilate with bag and mask until the required equipment or expertise is to hand. The commonest cause of cardiac arrest in children is not primary heart disease but hypoxia.

BASIC LIFE SUPPORT

Airway

The tongue is large and a degree of obstruction from this and enlarged adenoids may already be present. A roll of towel or sandbag should be placed under the shoulders and the jaw lifted forward with a finger behind the mandible. The airway must be held with the fingers supporting only bony structures. Pressure on soft tissues in the floor of the mouth will only increase the obstruction.

Check that no foreign body is present in the mouth, (using forceps to remove it under direct vision if available).

- *Do not use blind finger-sweeps which may force the obstruction further into the airway.*

Breathing

Initially, a check should be made for foreign bodies or vomit and then exhaled air resuscitation (EAR) commenced unless a bag and mask is available.

Even opening the airway may allow the resumption of spontaneous ventilation. Assisted breathing may be required. The mouth and nose should be covered with one's own mouth in small infants, larger children should be ventilated with the nose pinched and one's own mouth applied to theirs.

Damage due to excessive tidal volume is unlikely but gastric distension is. Rapid, smaller breaths, sufficient to adequately expand the chest, are preferable. It is difficult in practice to achieve a rate much in excess of 25 breaths per minute, but this should be adequate.

Circulation

Circulatory arrest or inadequacy may occur with bradycardia following vagal stimulation as in, for example, the oculocardiac reflex. Hypoxia rapidly leads to profound bradycardia with no effective cardiac output. Cyanosis is rare in these circumstances. Children with congenital heart disease and right-to-left shunts may usually be cyanosed and in these children the sign is unhelpful in evaluating the situation. If no major pulses are palpable, a diagnosis of circulatory (cardiac) arrest is made. The brachial pulse is said to be easiest to feel in infants,[2] but the femoral is a good alternative.

Chest compression

Closed chest cardiac compression requires a different technique in small infants.[3] Both hands are placed around the child and the sternum compressed with both thumbs against the palms of the hands (see Fig. 14.1). It is vital not to cause abdominal compression and so pressure must only be applied to the sternum. The heart is centred under the lower third of the sternum in small[4] and larger[5] children. Cardiac compression should be carried out in a ratio of 5 compressions to 1 ventilation in infants and smaller children, even with one rescuer, and 15:2 in teenagers. Aim for a rate of 100 compressions per minute in infants *and* children.

Call for help

After one minute of basic life support help must be summoned. This may mean suspending resuscitation.

Choking (Fig. 14.2)

Sometimes an inhaled obstruction is not immediately suspected. If choking seems likely an artificial cough can be produced by:

- *back blows* — 5 sharp blows between the shoulder blades in a head-down, prone position.
- *chest thrusts*, again in a head-down position, but supine (similar to chest compressions, but more forceful at a rate of 20 min^{-1} (but 5 at a time — then re-open the airway and check breathing). In infants back blows and chest thrusts should be repeatedly alternated. In older children over 1 year of age 5 abdominal thrusts should be given after the second

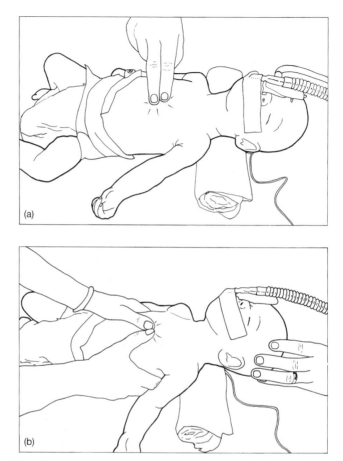

Fig. 14.1 Closed chest compression to assist circulation. (a) using finger tips (larger infants); (b) using thumbs (smaller infants).

sequence of back blows — upright (Heimlich manoeuvre) if conscious or supine if unconscious. (*Abdominal thrusts are not recommended in babies under 1 year of age because of risk of damage to the abdominal viscera.*)

ADVANCED LIFE SUPPORT TECHNIQUES

Intubation

When appropriate, intubation of the trachea should be accomplished by someone skilled in the technique. If mask ventilation is employed, the stomach should be drained through a gastric tube. If this interferes with the face mask seal, it can be done oro-gastrically, intermittently using a large bore tube each time gastric distension becomes apparent. The use of an oral airway of the Guedel type may improve the airway but frequently it does not

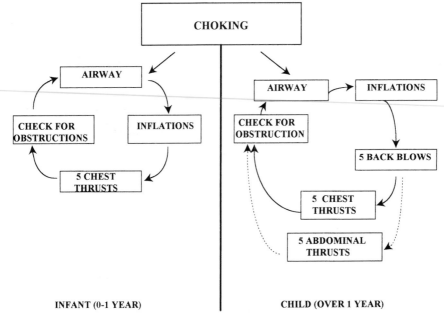

Fig. 14.2 Algorithm for management of choking.

as its shape is anatomically incorrect. The more curved 1A Guedel airway is rarely available. A nasopharyngeal airway may be more useful.

Endotracheal tube sizes and lengths can be swiftly determined by reference to Oakley's chart (Fig. 14.3). A full range must always be available with a selection of laryngoscopes. It is vital that frequent checks of resuscitation equipment be made and that all the components are assembled to ensure that they fit together. If self-inflating bags are used for ventilation (rather than an anaesthetic breathing system, such as a T-piece), the infant size should be equipped with a pressure-limiting blow-off valve which can be over-ridden if lung compliance is poor. Self-inflating bags require less skill in use than the T-piece circuit but it may be difficult to guarantee ventilation with 100 per cent oxygen, unless a reservoir bag is used which prevents all air entrainment.

Vascular access

In a collapsed baby, peripheral veins may be impossible to find. Good sites to try are the long saphenous vein or cubital fossa veins. Central venous cannulation provides guaranteed access but takes longer than intraosseous cannulation (see below) which should be carried out if venous access is not established within 90 sec.[1]

- *Central venous cannulation should be secondary to intraosseous access.* Scalp veins tend to 'blow-out' easily and are used as a last resort. The external

Endotrachael tube

Length (cm)	Internal diameter (mm)
18–21	75–80
18	7.0
17	6.5
16	6.0
15	5.5
14	5.0
13	4.5
12	4.0
	3.5
10	3.0–3.5

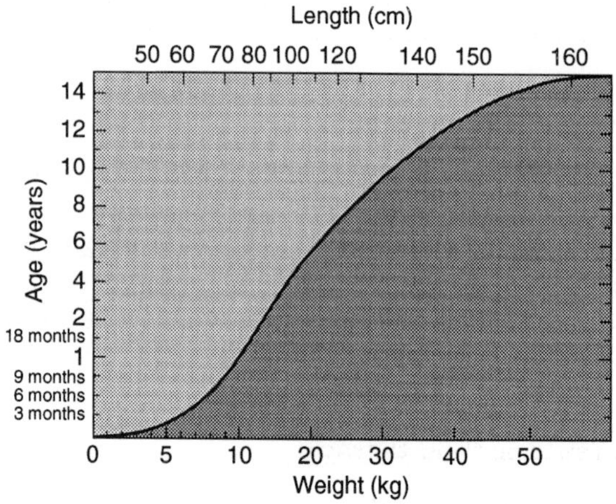

Fig. 14.3 Paediatric resuscitation chart. The graph represents age plotted against weight for the 50th centile boy-girl average. To the left are shown dimensions of endotracheal tubes, which correlate well with age. Adapted from Oakley, P. A. (1988). Inaccuracy and delay in decision making in paediatric resuscitation and a proposed reference chart to reduce error. *British Medical Journal*, 297, 1584.

jugular vein is easily visible but often very mobile and difficult to cannulate, especially in babies with their short necks.

Surgical cut-down can be used but takes much longer. It should only be considered if intraosseous access fails and expertise is not available to site an internal jugular, subclavian or femoral cannula.

Intra-osseous access

A study by Seigler *et al.*[6] has shown that fluid resuscitation or drug administration via the marrow space of the tibia or femur, first described in 1922,[7] is a suitable technique for use in pre-hospital care. Of 17 patients with cardiopulmonary arrest, 13 had an infusion established within 1 min and there were no significant complications.

Rossetti *et al.* found that 10 mins or longer was required to establish intravenous access in 25 per cent of 66 arrested paediatric patients.[8] The ease with which intra-osseous infusions can be established makes it a very attractive alternative a central cannulation. The mean time for surgical cut-down in Rossetti's paper is quoted as 24 mins. A recent case report highlights the usefulness of this technique in children.[9]

The intra-osseous needle is sited just below the tibial tuberosity if possible (see Fig. 14.4).

Haemoglobin concentration, electrolytes, glucose, venous pH and blood grouping can all be done as a marrow aspirate obtained when the intra-osseous needle is sited. Resuscitation drugs, fluid, and blood can be given by this route as the marrow cavity is contiguous with the rest of the circulation. *Fluids must, however, be given by pressure infusion (e.g. with a syringe).*

Other sites of access

Some drugs can successfully be given via the tracheal tube through a catheter into the bronchial-tree (adrenaline, atropine, lignocaine), although this is the least effective route. Studies indicate that ten times the intravenous dose of adrenaline is required.[10] Information on the effective doses of atropine or lignocaine is lacking. The intracardiac route should be avoided as myocardial damage and tamponade may occur.

Parenteral fluid therapy

In circulatory arrest due to hypovolaemia, volume replacement with a colloid, 0.9 per cent saline, or Hartmann's solution is appropriate but care

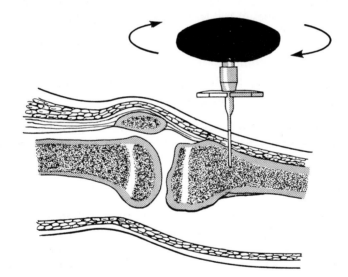

Fig. 14.4 Intraosseous needle insertion.

- The intraosseous needle should be inserted with a screwing motion into the marrow cavity (some needles or 'nails' have a self-tapping screw thread). The recommended sites are:
- anterior surface of tibia, 2 cm below tibial tuberosity
- anterolateral surface of femur, 3 cm above lateral condyle

Procedure
- clean skin
- insert needle at 90° to skin
- insert needle with screwing motion until loss of resistance is felt
- aspirate marrow with a syringe (send for Hb, U and E, cross-match)
- infuse fluid *under pressure* with 20 or 50 ml syringe attached to 3 way tap in giving set.

must be taken to avoid hypoglycaemia. In small children, 5 per cent dextrose with 0.9 per cent saline may be appropriate.

If hypovolaemia is not a feature, large sodium loads should be avoided. Even 1 mmol kg^{-1} sodium bicarbonate provides a considerable sodium load. Minimal volumes of 5 per cent or 10 per cent dextrose can be used but care must be taken not to precipitate or worsen cerebral oedema. If necessary 20 per cent glucose should be given slowly to treat hypoglycaemia and reduce the water load.

Animal experiments have shown that hyperglycaemia increases ischaemic brain injury.[11,12]

Resuscitation drugs

Even in paediatric medicine, doses are usually calculated on a per kilogram basis, although surface area equates better with extracellular fluid volume (see Chapter 2). In an emergency, the weight of a child can be guessed but is rarely known with accuracy, even by the parent. Rapid measurement of length with a tape-measure will allow calculation of endotracheal tube sizes and drug doses based on average length/weight relationships. A chart can be used to provide a quick reference for use in emergencies (Fig. 14.3).

Adrenaline is the commonest drug used to treat acute circulatory insufficiency in children. Oxygen alone may alleviate bradycardia due to hypoxia. One hundred per cent oxygen should always be used; the risk of retrolental fibroplasia or pulmonary toxicity is minimal and need not be considered during acute resuscitation.

Table 14.1 gives the doses of commonly used resuscitation drugs, together with their doses and indications.

DC SHOCK

Most cardiac arrests in children are adequately managed with drug therapy alone. Defibrillation is only rarely required for ventricular fibrillation or ventricular tachycardia. DC shock is sometimes used for other tachydysrhythmias refractory to drug therapy.

Excess energy can cause severe burns to the skin and myocardial damage. All the usual precautions for defibrillation of the patient must be observed.

DC shock must always be preceded by ventilation with 100 per cent oxygen.

The following are essential:
- correct paddle position (anterolateral; anteroposterior)
- good contact with low impedance (use of gel pads)
- adherence to protocols for correct energy selection

Table 14.1 Resuscitation drugs

Drug	Indication(s)	Dose	Route	Interaction or complications
Adrenaline	Asystole Hypotension due to pump failure	$5-10\ \mu g\ kg^{-1}$ $0.05-1.0\ \mu g\ kg^{-1}\ min^{-1}$ ($1\ mg = 1\ ml$ of 1 in 1000)	IV/IO (ET = dose $\times$ 10) IV infusion	Incompatible with bicarbonate
Atropine	Bradycardia 2nd and 3rd degree heart block Idioventricular rhythm	$5-20\ \mu g\ kg^{-1}$	IV/IO/ET	Large doses may cause tachydysrhythmia
Bicarbonate	Metabolic acidosis based on blood gas analysis. Full correction = (body wt $\times$ $0.3 \times$ base deficit) mmol. Often half correction only is required. Measure base deficit after half correction *NB. Arterial pH does not equate to tissue pH in cardiac arrest. Use MIXED VENOUS pH.*	$1\ mmol\ kg^{-1}$ maximum until pH and base deficit measured (*only give if first dose of adrenalin ineffective*)	IV	Extravascular infusion may lead to tissue necrosis, hypernatraemia and fluid overload, metabolic alkalosis, increased CO_2 production. Incompatible with adrenaline and other catecholamines or calcium salts
Calcium salts	To augment myocardial contractility Low ionized calcium	10% chloride $10\ mg\ kg^{-1}$ ($0.1\ ml\ kg^{-1}$) (preferred)	IV	Increase myocardial ischaemia and reperfusion injury

Table 14.1 (*continued*)

Drug	Indication(s)	Dose	Route	Interaction or complications
(*only indicated in cases of proven hypocalcaemia, hyperkalaemia, or hypermagnesaemia — NOT FOR ROUTINE USE*)		10% gluconate 30 mg kg^{-1} (0.3 ml kg^{-1})		Contraindicated in patients receiving cardiac glycosides
Dobutamine	Low cardiac output (tachycardia less evident than with dopamine)	5–10 μg kg^{-1} min^{-1} *Easy dose calculation:* *(3 × body weight)* *mg in 50 ml fluid* *1 ml h^{-1} = 1 μg kg^{-1} min^{-1}*	IV infusion	Hypertension Additive effect with other vasopressors
Dopamine	Low cardiac ouput	5–20 μg kg^{-1} min^{-1} by infusion	IV infusion	Hypertension Additive effect with other vasopressors
	Low urine output associated with hypotension	2–8 μg kg^{-1} min^{-1} *Easy dose calculation:* *(3 × body weight)* *mg in 50 ml fluid* *1 ml h^{-1} = 1 μg kg^{-1} min^{-1}*	IV infusion	

Table 14.1 (*continued*)

Drug	Indication(s)	Dose	Route	Interaction or complications
Ephedrine	Low cardiac output, low BP due to peripheral vasodilation	$0.1–0.4$ mg kg^{-1}	IV	Hypertension Additive effect with other vasopressors
Frusemide	Low urine output despite adequate fluid load	$0.5–1.0$ mg kg^{-1}	IV	Potassium depletion Ototoxicity
Isoprenaline	Bradycardia Bradydysrhythmia	1 μg kg^{-1} $0.01–0.5$ μg kg^{-1} min^{-1} (*30 μg kg in 50 ml fluid* *1 ml h^{-1} = 0.01 μg kg^{-1} min^{-1}*)	IV IV infusion	Tachycardia Hypertension Additive effect with other vasopressors
Lignocaine	Ventricular extrasystoles Tachydysrhythmias Refractory ventricular fibrillation (to precede DC shock) Infusion for recurrent extrasystoles	1 mg kg^{-1} 0.1 mg kg^{-1} min^{-1}	IV/IO IV infusion	CNS stimulation
Mannitol 20%	Forced diuresis for cerebral oedema	1 g kg^{-1} (5 ml kg^{-1})	IV infusion	Fluid overload Cardiac failure

IV = intravenous; IO = intraosseous; ET = endotracheal.

MANAGEMENT ALGORITHMS FOR DYSRHYTHMIA AND CARDIAC ARREST

Bradycardia

- Bradycardia in children is almost always due to hypoxia or hypoxia combined with low cardiac output.

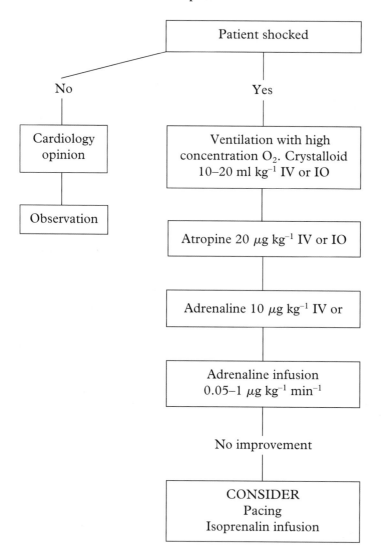

- $10\ \mu g\ kg^{-1}$ adrenaline = 0.1 ml kg^{-1} of 1:10 000 adrenaline

IV = intravenous
IO = intraosseous

Supraventricular tachycardia (SVT)

- This is rarely seen in children. Sinus tachycardia may be very fast in a baby (160 beats min^{-1} or more).

- If the child is not shocked, vagal manoeuvres such as immersion of the face in cold water (diving reflex) carotid sinus massage or a Valsalva manoeuvre (older children) can be tried.

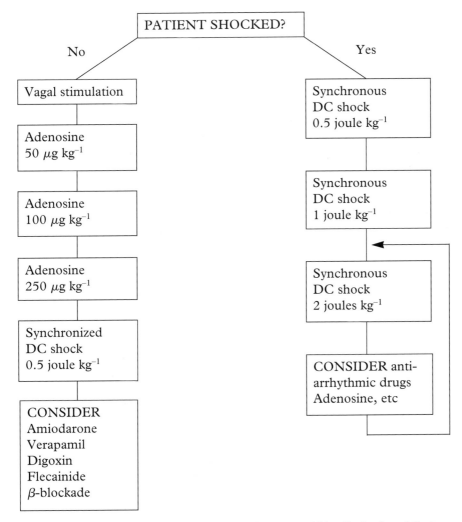

- NB. Adenosine has a very short half life. It should be flushed rapidly into a large vein.

- Do not give verapamil and β-blockers together.

- Verapamil is contraindicated in children under 1 year of age (risk of asystole).

Ventricular tachycardia

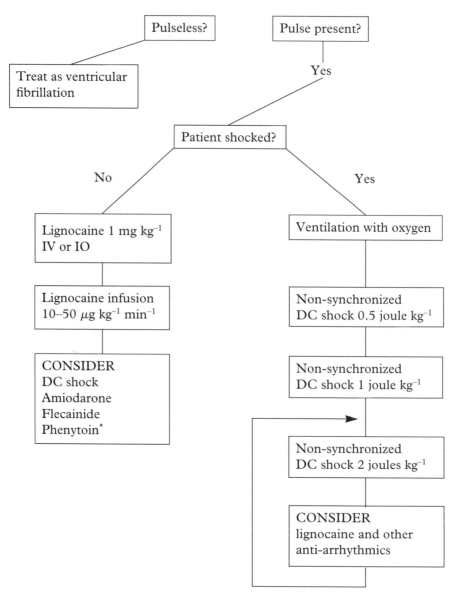

- Ventricular tachycardia may precede ventricular fibrillation or develop following successful defibrillation.
- * Phenytoin is particularly indicated in dysrhythmia due to tricyclic overdose.

IV = intravenous

IO = intraosseous

Asystole

- This is the commonest cause of cardiac arrest in children. *It is almost always due to hypoxia.*
- Good basic life support technique is essential.

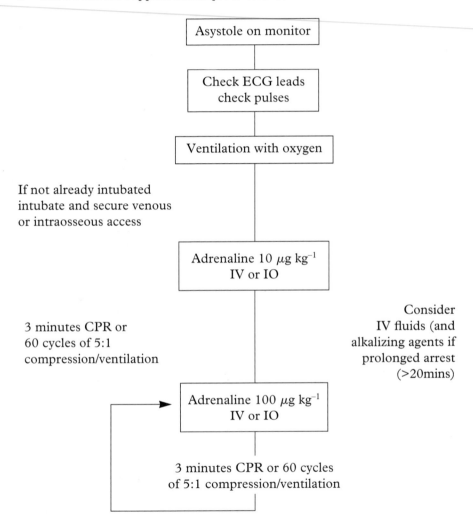

	Asystole on monitor
	Check ECG leads / check pulses
	Ventilation with oxygen

If not already intubated intubate and secure venous or intraosseous access

Adrenaline 10 μg kg^{-1} IV or IO

3 minutes CPR or 60 cycles of 5:1 compression/ventilation

Consider IV fluids (and alkalizing agents if prolonged arrest (>20mins)

Adrenaline 100 μg kg^{-1} IV or IO

3 minutes CPR or 60 cycles of 5:1 compression/ventilation

- 10 μg kg^{-1} = 0.1 ml kg^{-1} of 1:10 000 adrenaline
- 100 μg kg^{-1} = 1 ml kg^{-1}of 1: 10 000 adrenaline
- Intraosseous drugs must be well flushed in with saline.

CPR = cardio pulmonary resuscitation
IV = intravenous
IO = intraosseous

Ventricular fibrillation (VF)

VF is uncommon in childhood cardiac arrests, but occurs in:

- hypothermia
- tricyclic overdose
- primary heart disease (rare)

- *Good basic life support is essential*

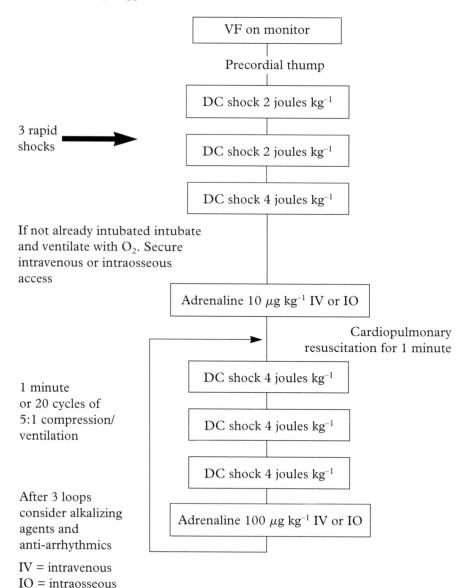

VF on monitor

Precordial thump

DC shock 2 joules kg^{-1}

3 rapid shocks ➤ DC shock 2 joules kg^{-1}

DC shock 4 joules kg^{-1}

If not already intubated intubate and ventilate with O_2. Secure intravenous or intraosseous access

Adrenaline 10 μg kg^{-1} IV or IO

Cardiopulmonary resuscitation for 1 minute

1 minute or 20 cycles of 5:1 compression/ ventilation

DC shock 4 joules kg^{-1}

DC shock 4 joules kg^{-1}

DC shock 4 joules kg^{-1}

After 3 loops consider alkalizing agents and anti-arrhythmics

Adrenaline 100 μg kg^{-1} IV or IO

IV = intravenous
IO = intraosseous

Electromechanical dissociation

- Hypovolaemia or tamponade may occur following traffic accidents.
- Drug overdose should always be considered.
- Pneumothorax is common in ventilated small babies.

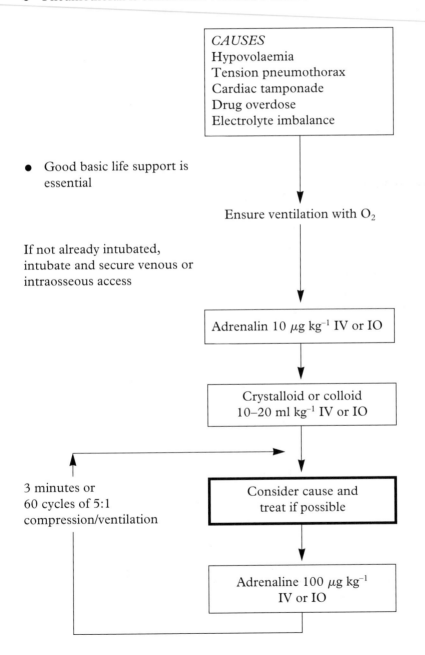

CAUSES
Hypovolaemia
Tension pneumothorax
Cardiac tamponade
Drug overdose
Electrolyte imbalance

- Good basic life support is essential

Ensure ventilation with O_2

If not already intubated, intubate and secure venous or intraosseous access

Adrenalin 10 μg kg^{-1} IV or IO

Crystalloid or colloid
10–20 ml kg^{-1} IV or IO

3 minutes or
60 cycles of 5:1
compression/ventilation

Consider cause and
treat if possible

Adrenaline 100 μg kg^{-1}
IV or IO

Post-resuscitation care

If resuscitation is successful and the patient is stable he should be transferred to an intensive care unit or high dependency area. Close observation is mandatory.

Essential monitoring consists of:

- ECG
- oxygen saturation
- blood pressure (preferably invasive)
- urine output and fluid balance
- core and skin temperatures
- acid–base status and blood gases (*arterial pH is not a good guide to tissue pH following cardiac arrest and the mixed venous pH is preferable*)

In addition capnography and cardiac output measurement may be useful.

> **It is recommended that all anaesthetists dealing with children should undergo training on an Advanced Paediatric Life Support Course (APLS)**

The protocols given in this chapter are consistent with the recommendations of the European Resuscitation Council. For a review of paediatric cardiopulmonary resuscitation the reader is referred to Richmond and Bingham.[13]

NEONATAL RESUSCITATION

Resuscitation in the delivery suite has become a well-organized and practised procedure. Asphyxia or trauma from a difficult delivery may be anticipated sufficiently in advance for expert help to be at hand immediately.

Assessment

Since the early 1960s the Apgar score has been the most widely used scoring system, certainly in the UK (see Table 14.2). The normal score is 8–10. Less significance is placed upon the infant's colour and the 'Apgar Minus Colour' score has sometimes been used.

Moderate asphyxia will result in an Apgar score of 4–7, severe asphyxia being indicated by a score of 0–3.

Table 14.2 Assessment for neonatal resuscitation using Apgar Score

Observation	Apgar Score		
	0	1	2
Heart rate	Absent	Less than 100	Greater than 100
Respiratory effort	Absent	Weak (gasping)	Crying
Muscle tone	Flaccid	Some flexion of limbs, no active movement	Well flexed, active movement
Reflex irritability	Nil	Grimace	Cough or sneeze
Colour	Pale or blue	Body pink, extremities blue	Overall pink

Record at 1 min and 5 mins after birth and at each 5 mins of continuing resuscitation.

Resuscitation is required if the heart rate is less than 100 beats min^{-1} and the baby is apnoeic or has a poor respiratory effort. *Resuscitation should not be delayed in order to assess an Apgar score.*

Primary apnoea

- the baby is blue
- has some muscle tone
- heart rate greater than 80 beats min^{-1}
- apnoeic or gasping

Terminal apnoea

- the baby is white rather than blue
- heart rate less than 80 beats min^{-1}
- apnoeic

Some babies are of course 'born dead' (fresh stillbirth). Such babies are:

- white
- pulseless
- apnoeic

Full cardiopulmonary resuscitation is justified if fetal monitoring indicated a live baby prior to delivery. Many babies make a full recovery. Unless there is a rapid response to resuscitation (spontaneous ventilation and cardiac output within 10 minutes) only a very few babies will survive. In this case the incidence of hypoxic brain damage (cerebral palsy) will be very high.
There may be a history of:

- antepartum haemorrhage (leading to severe asphyxia)

- bleeding from the umbilical cord
- meconium aspiration (see below)
- prematurity (resuscitation more likely to be required)

Management

Prevention of heat loss

Prevention of heat loss is achieved by immediate drying and swaddling, use of radiant heat or a foil blanket. Cold stress vastly increases oxygen requirements.

Airway

Care should be taken during suction of meconium or liquor not to pass the catheter beyond the oropharynx as severe bradycardia may ensue. If apnoea persists beyond 1 min, the baby should be transferred to a resuscitation trolley or firm surface under a radiant heater if possible, or well-wrapped in a dry towel. The infant should be slightly head-up or horizontal to allow good diaphragmatic excursion. For Apgar score 4–7 the infant may be stimulated by flicking the soles of the feet or with an oxygen jet on the skin.

For babies with primary apnoea, positive pressure ventilation with oxygen or oxygen-enriched air may be required. Some babies will respond to high flow oxygen alone. Those with terminal apnoea need positive pressure ventilation. Bag and mask using a manometer or blow-off valve (max 30 cm H_2O) is often sufficient. *Intubation is not required unless bag and mask is unsuccessful within 1 min. In mildly asphyxiated babies, intubation may cause severe reflex stimulation and do more harm than good.*

Once respiration is established, the baby must not be left to breathe through an endotracheal tube unless continuous positive airway pressure (CPAP) is applied (see Chapter 1). The tube should be removed as soon as regular respiration is established. If the mother has received any opioid drugs within 12 h of birth, the baby should receive naloxone 40 μg kg^{-1} intramuscularly (intravenous access will not be available easily except via the umbilical vein). Effective plasma levels are achieved within 5 min provided muscle blood flow is adequate.

Circulation

Bradycardia of less than 100 beats min^{-1} despite adequate ventilation, lack of heart sounds, or undetectable apex beat require chest compression. Both hands are placed around the chest and the thumbs used to compress the lower sternum at a rate of not less than 100 per minute. Persistent circulatory failure should be treated according to the protocol for asystole.

Drugs should be given into the umbilical vein and flushed in.

Sodium bicarbonate is contraindicated unless a severe metabolic acidosis is shown on blood gas estimation. If blood gas analysis is not available 1 mmol kg^{-1} may be given after 20 mins of circulatory arrest in an attempt to improve the efficacy of the adrenaline.

Further management points

During resuscitation with intermittent positive pressure ventilation (IPPV), one must continuously be alert to the possibility of pneumothorax.

Failed resuscitation may be due to a severe congenital anomaly such as diaphragmatic hernia, congenital heart disease, anencephaly, cerebrospinal malformation, or congenital lobar emphysema. Pneumothorax must be excluded.

The presence of meconium should alert one to the possibility of meconium aspiration. This condition is associated with atelectasis and persistent fetal circulatory pattern. It can largely be prevented by meticulous management at delivery. The mouth, nose, and pharynx should be aspirated under direct vision while the chest is held compressed to prevent gasping. *IPPV must not be used before clearing the airway.*

Blood loss

Fetal blood loss may occur at delivery, necessitating blood transfusion (matched against mother's blood or with O-negative blood).

REFERENCES

1. Paediatric Life Support Working Party of the European Resuscitation Council (1994). Guidelines for paediatric life support. *British Medical Journal*, **308**, 1349.
2. Cavallaro, D. L. and Melter, R. J. (1983). Comparison of two techniques for detecting cardiac activity in infants. *Critical Care Medicine*, **11**, 190.
3. Thaler, M. M. and Stobie, G. H. C. (1963). An improved technique of external cardiac compression in infants and young children. *New England Journal of Medicine*, **269**, 606.
4. Phillips, G. W. L. and Zideman, D. A. (1986). Relation of the infant heart to the sternum: its significance in cardiopulmonary resuscitation. *Lancet*, **i**, 1024.
5. Orlowski, U. P. (1986). Optimum position for external cardiac compression in infants and young children. *Annals of Emergency Medicine*, **15**, 667.
6. Seigler, R. S., Techlenbury, F. E., and Shealy, R. (1989). Prehospital intraosseous infusion by emergency medical services personnel: a prospective study. *Pediatrics*, **84**, 173.
7. Drinker, C. K., Drinker, K. R., and Lund, C. C. (1922). Circulation in mammalian bone marrow with especial reference concerned in movement of red blood cells from bone marrow into circulation blood as disclosed by perfusion of tibia of dog and by injections of bone marrow in rabbit and cat. *American Journal of Physiology*, **62**, 1.
8. Rossetti, V. *et al.* (1984). Difficulty and delay in intravenous access in pediatric arrest. *Annals of Emergency Medicine*, **13**, 406.
9. Gibson, M., Clancy, M. J., and Illingworth, R. N. (1990). Intraosseous infusion for emergency vascular access in children. *British Journal of Accident and Emergency Medicine*, **5**, 11.

10. Quinton, D. N., O'Byrne, G., and Aitkenhead , A. R. (1987). Comparison of endotracheal and peripheral venous intravenous adrenaline in cardiac arrest: is the endotracheal route reliable? *Lancet*, (1987) **(i)**, 828.
11. Pulsinelli, W. A., Waldman, S., Rawlinson, D. *et al.* (1982). Moderate hyperglycaemia augments ischaemic brain damage: a neuropathologic study in the rat. *Neurology*, **32**, 1239.
12. Nakakimura, K., Fleischer, J. E., Drummond, J. C. *et al.* (1990). Glucose administration before cardiac arrest worsens neurologic outcome in cats. *Anesthesiology*, **72**, 1005.
13. Richmond, C. E. and Bingham, R. M. (1995). Paediatric cardiopulmonary resuscitation. *Paediatric Anaesthesia*, **5**, 11.

Appendix 1

Guidelines for fluid maintenance requirements

Weight (kg)	Fluid per 24 h (ml kg^{-1})	Fluid per hour (ml kg^{-1})
Up to 10	100	4
Next 10	50	2
Subsequent kg	20	1

For example, a child weighing 27 kg requires:

For first 10 kg	$10 \times 100 = 1000$ ml
For next 10 kg	$10 \times 50 = 500$ ml
For remaining 7 kg	$7 \times 20 = 140$ ml

Total	1640 ml in 24 h

Appendix 2

Table of endotracheal tube sizes

Age	Weight (kg)	Internal diameter (mm)	Length (cm)
Premature	2.5 or less	2.5–3.0	8.5–9.0
Neonate	3.0	3.0–3.5	9.0–9.5
6 months	6.0	4.0	10–11.0
1 year	10.0	4.5	12.0
2 years	12–13.0	5.0	13.0
3	14–15.0	5.0	13.5
4	16.0	5.5	14.0
5	18.0	5.5	14.5
6	20.0	6.0	15.0
7	22.0	6.0	15.5
8	24.0	6.5	16.0
9	26–28.0	6.5	16.5
10	30–32.0	7.0	17.0
11	32–34.0	7.0	17.5
12	36.0	7.5	18.0
13	40.0	7.5	18.5
14	45.0+	8.0	19.0
15	50.0+	8.0	20.0

- These sizes are only a guide. Considerable individual variation exists. Tube length is more closely related to age than weight.
- Armoured tubes have thicker walls than standard PVC tubes and so one size smaller than indicated in the chart may be required.

Appendix 3

Recommended doses of some commonly used drugs

Note that these dosages are only intended as guidelines. Before prescribing any drug you should consult the most recent edition of the *British National Formulary* or follow the manufacturer's instructions.

NB   THESE DOSES MAY BE INAPPROPRIATE FOR NEONATES

Induction agents

Ketamine	1–2 mg kg^{-1} IV; 10 mg kg^{-1} IM.
Methohexitone	1–2 mg kg^{-1} IV.
Propofol	2.5–3.5 mg kg^{-1} IV.
Thiopentone	5–6 mg kg^{-1} IV.

Muscle relaxants — initial dose

Atracurium	0.5–0.6 mg kg^{-1} IV. 0.5 mg kg^{-1} h^{-1} by IV infusion.
Mivacurium	0.15–0.2 mg kg^{-1} IV.
Pancuronium	0.1–0.15 mg kg^{-1} IV.
Suxamethonium	1–2 mg kg^{-1} IV.
d-tubocurarine	0.5 mg kg^{-1} IV.
Vecuronium	0.1 mg kg h^{-1} by IV infusion.

Analgesics

Opioids

*Alfentanil	10–50 μg kg^{-1} IV as required. 20–60 μg kg^{-1} h^{-1} by IV infusion (loading dose 50–100 μg kg^{-1}).

Buprenorphine	3–6 mg kg^{-1} sublingual 6–8 hourly.
Codeine phosphate	1 mg kg^{-1} IM 4–6 hourly.
	(NB *Not to be given intravenously.*)
*Fentanyl	1–10 μg kg^{-1} IV as required (loading dose for infusion 2–5 μg kg^{-1}).
	(Up to 100 μg kg^{-1} if post-operative ventilation is planned.)
	2–8 μg kg^{-1} h^{-1} by IV infusion.
*Morphine	0.15–0.2 mg kg^{-1} 2–4 hourly IV or IM
	10–40 μg kg^{-1} by IV infusion.
Nalbuphine	0.3 mg kg^{-1} 3–4 hourly IV or IM.
Pethidine	1–2 mg kg^{-1} 2–4 hourly IV or IM.

NB   Infusion dose depends upon loading dose and presence of other opioids (infusion doses will usually be inadequate unless a loading dose is given).

Caution: RESPIRATORY DEPRESSION MAY BE PROFOUND FOLLOWING INFUSION OF OPIOIDS.

Opioid reversal

Administration of intravenous naloxone (Narcan)

- Take one vial of naloxone 400 μg ml^{-1} and draw up into 10 ml syringe.
- Add 9 ml of 0.9% NaCl to provide a solution of 40 μg ml^{-1}. (For babies less than 10 kg, repeat the dilution to give a final solution of 4 μg ml^{-1}).
- Carefully titrate 1 μg kg^{-1} of naloxone intravenously every two to three minutes until respiratory rate or conscious level satisfactory.
- Effective response = reversal of respiratory depression, minimal to moderate reversal of sedation, and *no reversal of analgesia*.
- Too much naloxone can result in vomiting, hypertension and severe pain.
- Observe closely — re narcotization may occur swiftly. The duration of action of naloxone is very short (maximum 20 minutes as given above).
- An infusion of naloxone may be required dose range: 3–10 μg kg h^{-1} initially, titrated according to response.

Non-opioid analgesics

| Paracetamol | 12–15 mg kg^{-1} oral or rectal 4–6 hourly (maximum dose 60 mg kg^{-1} 24 h^{-1}). |

Non-steroidal anti-inflammatory analgesics

| Diclofenac | 1–1.5 mg kg^{-1} oral or rectal. (maximum dose 3 mg kg^{-1} 24h^{-1}) |

| | (A dispersible oral preparation is available which facilitates correct oral dosing) |
| Ibuprofen | Paediatric elixir (20 mg ml^{-1} dose 5 mg kg^{-1}) 200 mg tablets (maximum dose 20 mg kg^{-1} 24 h^{-1} in 4 divided doses). |

Benzodiazepines

Premedication	Oral	Temazepam 0.5–1 mg kg^{-1} to maximum 30 mg
	Oral	Diazepam 0.5–1 mg kg^{-1} to maximum 30 mg.
Sedation	IV	Diazepam 0.1–0.25 mg kg^{-1} by incremental bolus. Infusion is *not* recommended. Midazolam loading dose of 0.15–0.2 mg kg^{-1}. Infusion 0.1–0.2 mg kg^{-1} h^{-1}.

Chloral derivatives

| Premedication short-term sedation | Oral | Chloral hydrate 30–50 mg kg^{-1} 6–8 hourly. |
| | Oral | Triclofos 50–100 mg kg^{-1} 6–8 hourly |

Local analgesic agents

	Without adrenalin	*With adrenalin 1:200 000*
Bupivacaine	3	4
Lignocaine	6	9
Prilocaine	6	–

NB. *Reduce dose of local anaesthetics in neonates.*

Reversal of neuromuscular block

| Neostigmine | 50 μg kg^{-1} IV |

When used with neostigmine

| Atropine | 20 μg kg^{-1} |
| Glycopyrronium (glycopyrrolate) | 10 μg kg^{-1} |

Appendix 3

Table of infusion regimens

Drug	Dilution	1 ml h^{-1} delivers:	Recommended dose range
Adrenaline	300 μg kg^{-1} in 50 ml	100 ng kg^{-1} min^{-1}	100–1000 ng kg^{-1} min^{-1}
Aminophyline	50 mg kg^{-1} in 50 ml	1 mg kg^{-1} hour^{-1}	0.5–1 mg kg h^{-1}
Atracurium	5 mg kg^{-1} in 50 ml	100 μg kg^{-1} h^{-1}	300–600 μg kg h^{-1}
Dobutamine	3 mg kg^{-1} in 50 ml	1 μg kg^{-1} min^{-1}	3–20 μg kg^{-1} min^{-1}
Dopamine	3 mg kg^{-1} in 50 ml	1 μg kg^{-1} hour^{-1}	3–20 μg kg^{-1} min^{-1}
Fentanyl	50 μg kg^{-1} in 50 ml	1 μg kg^{-1} hour^{-1}	2–4 μg^{-1} kg^{-1} h^{-1}
Isoprenaline	300 μg kg^{-1} in 50 ml	100 ng kg^{-1} min^{-1}	20–200 ng kg^{-1} min^{-1}
Morphine	0.5 mg kg^{-1} in 50 ml	10 μg kg^{-1} hour^{-1}	5–40 μg kg^{-1} h^{-1}
Midazolam★	5 mg kg^{-1} in 50 ml	100 μg kg^{-1} hour^{-1}	50–300 μg kg^{-1} h^{-1}
Nitroglycerin★★	3 mg kg^{-1} in 50 ml	1 μg kg^{-1} min^{-1}	200–1000 ng kg^{-1} min^{-1}
Nitroprusside★★★	3 mg kg^{-1} in 50 ml	1 μg kg^{-1} min^{-1}	0.3–1.5 μg kg^{-1} min^{-1}
Noradrenaline	300 μg kg^{-1} in 50 ml	100 ng kg^{-1} min^{-1}	100–1000 ng kg^{-1} min^{-1}
Prostaglandin E2	15 μg kg^{-1} in 50 ml	5 ng kg^{-1} min^{-1}	5–20 ng kg^{-1} min^{-1}
Prostacyclin★★★★	15 μg kg^{-1} in 50 ml	5 ng kg^{-1} min^{-1}	5–20 ng kg^{-1} min^{-1}
Tolazoline	50 mg kg^{-1} in 50 ml	1 mg kg^{-1} hour^{-1}	1–2 mg kg^{-1} h^{-1}
Vecuronium	5 mg kg^{-1} in 50 ml	100 μg kg^{-1} hour^{-1}	50–100 μg kg^{-1} h^{-1}

> 1 mg = 1000 μg   1 μg = 1000 nanograms (ng)

NB   For most drugs an initial *LOADING DOSE* will be required.

★   Midazolam infusion maximum concentration 2 mg ml^{-1} (25 mg in 50 ml).

★★   Nitroglycerin maximum concentration 1 mg ml^{-1} (50 mg in 50 ml). (Can be given undiluted if absolutely necessary because of fluid restriction
NB. Avoid PVC tubing and giving sets — polyethylene tubing is suitable.)

★★★   Nitroprusside infusions must be protected from light.

★★★★   Prostacyclin minimum concentration 70 μg in 50 ml.

Index